# Recent Advances in Geriatric Medicine

## *(Volume 2)*

### *(An Interdisciplinary Approach to Geriatric Medicine)*

## Edited by

## Jeremy W. Grabbe

*Department of Psychology, The State University of New York, Plattsburgh*
*101 Broad St., Plattsburgh, NY 12801, USA*

liability of Bentham Science Publishers shall be limited to the amount actually paid by you for the Work.

## General:

1. Any dispute or claim arising out of or in connection with this License Agreement or the Work (including non-contractual disputes or claims) will be governed by and construed in accordance with the laws of the U.A.E. as applied in the Emirate of Dubai. Each party agrees that the courts of the Emirate of Dubai shall have exclusive jurisdiction to settle any dispute or claim arising out of or in connection with this License Agreement or the Work (including non-contractual disputes or claims).
2. Your rights under this License Agreement will automatically terminate without notice and without the need for a court order if at any point you breach any terms of this License Agreement. In no event will any delay or failure by Bentham Science Publishers in enforcing your compliance with this License Agreement constitute a waiver of any of its rights.
3. You acknowledge that you have read this License Agreement, and agree to be bound by its terms and conditions. To the extent that any other terms and conditions presented on any website of Bentham Science Publishers conflict with, or are inconsistent with, the terms and conditions set out in this License Agreement, you acknowledge that the terms and conditions set out in this License Agreement shall prevail.

**Bentham Science Publishers Ltd.**
Executive Suite Y - 2
PO Box 7917, Saif Zone
Sharjah, U.A.E.
Email: subscriptions@benthamscience.org

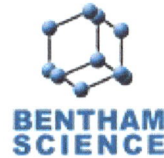

# CONTENTS

# PREFACE

This eBook will provide a one-of-its-kind comprehensive examination of recent advances in geriatric medicine. The field of geriatric medicine has expanded exponentially in recent decades due to the increase of the world-wide aging population. According to the National Institute of Aging (www.nia.nih.gov) there are now more than half a billion people over the age of 65 across the globe. This has led to an increase in the need for medical and psychiatric care on a scale unprecedented in history. In light of this change in the population the field of geriatric medicine has become multidisciplinary.

One of the unfortunate consequences of a large multidisciplinary field is that advances that occur within a specific discipline are not always readily conveyed to the other disciplines within geriatric medicine. The growth of highly-specialized journals has made research and advances far more insular. Because of this insular nature within disciplines there have been more problems in large complex settings such as nursing homes which utilize varied professionals of geriatric health.

This eBook will provide a novel approach by highlighting recent advances in geriatric medicine across different disciplines. This will enable clinicians not just to understand what new treatments/discoveries there are, but to allow them the comprehensive understanding necessary to work as a team in a new 21$^{st}$ century approach to geriatric medicine.

Another point where this eBook will break ground on new important issues is the approach it will take in providing insight into the various living conditions of older adults. As the aging population increases so do the diverse living conditions of older adults increase as well. Large numbers of older adults are living independently within the community. However, the population in assisted living residences and nursing homes is increasing. The ability of older adults to contribute to their well-being and interaction with health care professionals is directly linked to their housing situation.

This eBook will attempt to provide a thorough and pervasive cross-section of this issue in order to provide the audience with a versatile understanding of each issue and how it is affected by older adults' housing circumstances. The diverse array of fields that are addressed in this book along with the broad issues, from dementia to stroke to physical therapy, will provide a valuable reference for the next generation of professionals.

## DEDICATION

For Lisa who helped me to stayed up late and for Regina, Alexander, and Daniella who woke me up early.

**Dr. Jeremy W. Grabbe**
The State University of New York, Plattsburgh
101 Broad St. Plattsburgh
NY 12901, USA

# List of Contributors

**Ann McCarthy**          John Carroll University, 1 John Carroll Blvd, University Heights, OH 44118, USA

**Caitlin Murphy**        The State University of New York, Plattsburgh, 101 Broad St. Plattsburgh, NY 12901, USA

**Daniela Fabiani-Longo**  The State University of New York, Plattsburgh, 101 Broad St. Plattsburgh, NY 12901, USA

**James Mullen**          The State University of New York, Plattsburgh, 101 Broad St. Plattsburgh, NY 12901, USA

**Jeremy W. Grabbe**      The State University of New York, Plattsburgh, 101 Broad St. Plattsburgh, NY 12901, USA

**Jesselee Allen**        The State University of New York, Plattsburgh, 101 Broad St. Plattsburgh, NY 12901, USA

**Jocelyn Dismore**       The State University of New York, Plattsburgh, 101 Broad St. Plattsburgh, NY 12901, USA

**Kate Hood**             Sunnyview Rehabilitation Hospital, 1270 Belmont Ave, Schenectady, NY 12308, USA

**Kathyrn McGeoch**       The State University of New York, Plattsburgh, 101 Broad St. Plattsburgh, NY 12901, USA

**Kayla Bishop**          The State University of New York, Plattsburgh, 101 Broad St. Plattsburgh, NY 12901, USA

**Paul D. Loprinzi**      The University of Mississippi, University, MS 38677, USA

**Rashmita Basu**         Texas A & M Health Science Center 8447 TX-47, Bryan, TX 77807, USA

**Robert E. Davis**       The University of Mississippi, University, MS 38677, USA

**Susan E. Lowey**        State University of New York College at Brockport, 350 New Campus Dr, Brockport, NY 14420, USA

**Tamara Pobocik**        The State University of New York, Plattsburgh 101 Broad St. Plattsburgh, NY 12901, USA

**Virginia Cornelius**    The State University of New York, Plattsburgh, 101 Broad St. Plattsburgh, NY 12901, USA

Recent Advances in Geriatric Medicine

# Recent Advances in Geriatric Medicine

## (Volume 2)

## (An Interdisciplinary Approach to Geriatric Medicine)

2

# Recent Advances in Geriatric Medicine

*Volume # 2*

*An Interdisciplinary Approach to Geriatric Medicine*

Editor:  Jeremy W. Grabbe

eISBN (Online): 978-1-68108-451-0

ISBN (Print): 978-1-68108-452-7

eISSN (Online): 2468-225X

ISSN (Print): 2468-2241

First published in 2017.

## CHAPTER 1

# The Basis of Geriatric Medicine

Jeremy W. Grabbe[*]

*The State University of New York, Plattsburgh 101 Broad St. Plattsburgh, NY 12901, USA*

**Abstract:** The study of aging and geriatrics is a relatively recent area of study and specialization. Much of the increase in focus on geriatrics has been a result of the explosion of the aging population. It therefore has become essential for the modern clinician to have an understanding of the different disciplines involved in administering to the aging population. Keeping track of recent advances can be a daunting undertaking. This chapter will prepare the reader to appreciate the multidisciplinary approach to geriatric medicine. This growing demographic has a dramatic impact on the future of scientific research.

**Keywords:** Aging population, Biogerontology, Geriatric medicine, History of geriatrics, Multidisciplinary approach, Research, Theories of aging.

## HISTORY OF GERIATRIC MEDICINE

Due to a relatively small population of older adults throughout history geriatrics was not particularly studied in detail. It was not until the 20th century that breakthroughs in medicine and advances in health, occupational safety, and standards of living allowed for the explosive increase of the older adult population. In 1909, the word "geriatrics" was first coined by Ignatz Nascher. In 1909, the average life expectancy in the U.S. was 52.2 years. It was nearly 25 years after Nascher coined the word geriatrics that the average life expectancy in the U.S. crossed over 60 years of age.

In the 1970s, greater interest in geriatrics bloomed. It became a focus for researchers and clinicians. In 1974, the National Institute on Aging was founded (incidentally the average U.S. life expectancy in 1974 was 72.1 years of age). In an interesting comparison, the field of geriatrics blossomed in the U.K. soon after the end of WWII (substantially earlier than the U.S.). However, the increase in life expectancy in the U.K. was remarkably similar to the increase in life

[*] **Corresponding author Jeremy W. Grabbe:** The State University of New York, Plattsburgh 101 Broad St. Plattsburgh, NY 12901, USA; Tel: 1(518) 792-5425; E-mail: jgrab001@plattsburgh.edu

expectancy in the U.S. throughout the 20<sup>th</sup> century. It can be speculated that the U.K. was proactive in anticipating the needs of the older adult population. Conversely, it could be assumed that the U.S. was slower to respond to the increasing older adult population.

In the 1980s, fellowships for physicians in geriatrics increased dramatically. The field of psychology saw a renewed interest in aging and brain function/behavior. The psychological community avoid the field of aging due to the negative implications of aging research that stemmed from G. Stanly Hall's 1922 book *Senescence*. These changes in medicine and psychology reflect advances in geriatric nursing in the previous decades. During the 1960s and 70s, nursing formalized geriatric nursing and joined the forefront of geriatrics. In the 21<sup>st</sup> century, the rise in the population of older adults has made geriatrics a factor in all branches of medicine and clinical practice. In fact, many clinicians find that the majority of patients are over the age of 65. Now is the time of the geriatrician.

## BASIS OF AGING

Currently, many theories exist to explain aging and the disorders common to aging. Many theories are specific to one particular aspect of aging. There are some pan-aging theories. In the subsequent chapters there will be more elaborate discussions of such theories. It becomes more imperative that different clinicians and researchers have an understanding of how recent advances influence new theory-based approaches to treatment.

For example, the Third Congress on Biogerontology [1] identified seven different points and prediction upon the soma theory and its role in modern geriatrics:

1. Ageing results from the gradual accumulation of damage in somatic cells and tissues and accordingly longevity is regulated by the efficacy of somatic maintenance and repair. This is now confirmed by a wide range of experimental studies, including comparative studies on repair capacity and stress resistance.
2. Germline immortality may be secured by enhanced mechanisms for maintenance and repair of germ cells, a strong example of this being the action of telomerase. Stem cells occupy an interesting position between germ- line and terminally differentiated somatic cells, and there is interesting data beginning to accumulate on intrinsic ageing of tissue stem cells, such as those of intestinal epithelium.
3. Trade-offs are predicted to exist between key life-history traits such as fertility and longevity, a prediction shared with the pleiotropy theory developed by

George Williams. There are many documented instances where such trade-offs have been observed but there are also some intriguing examples where the existence of trade- offs is yet to be demonstrated.

4. Since the central mechanism of ageing is predicted to be the accumulation of random molecular damage, a key prediction is that the ageing process is inherently stochastic. There is growing evidence to support this and it appears likely that further studies on the role of intrinsic chance variations in ageing will be necessary in order to understand the variability of the senescent phenotype.

5. Multiple, complex systems contribute to the underlying causes of ageing. This requires the development and application of new 'systems biology' methods, including in silico models, in order to address the potential synergism between different candidate mechanisms.

6. The theory predicts that ageing results from evolutionary optimisation of the life history, subject to a number of intrinsic and extrinsic constraints imposed by ecological and physiological factors. This provides a series of interesting problems in terms of understanding how optimality principles have helped to shape organisms' life cycles.

7. The theory suggests that there may be significant opportunity for organisms to have evolved plastic responses to allow them to cope with variable environmental conditions. A good example is the calorie-restriction response in rodents, which the disposable soma theory suggests might have its origins in evolving a plastic response to periods of interrupted food supply.

## FUTURE DIRECTIONS

One new and rather germane topic currently in discussion is just who is a geriatrician [2]? This discussion originated as the global population of older adults continued to expand. Now clinicians must cope with a diverse array of older adults as well as conditions and factors. Questions to be asked are what type of population should be the focus: community-dwelling or assisted-living? Young-old or old-old? Chronological age or functional age? Clearly this is not a debate that can be settled in one session let alone one book. The goal of this book is to discuss recent advances in the treatment and interactions with the geriatric population.

As the geriatric population becomes diverse so do the people who work with and study older adults. This book attempts to elucidate on the myriad of different disciplines currently involved in geriatrics. In this book physicians, academics, scientists as well as speech-language pathologists, physical therapists, and the cornerstone of care, nursing (among other disciplines), address the advances and new areas of interest in these broad fields. This will provide the reader with a greater appreciation of the interdisciplinary field of geriatric medicine.

## CONFLICT OF INTEREST

The author confirms that author has no conflict of interest to declare for this publication.

## ACKNOWLEDGEMENTS

Declared none.

## REFERENCES

[1]   Bergamini E. The third European congress on biogerontology: the biogerontological basis of preventive medicine and geriatric practice. Exp Gerontol 2003; 38(10): 1213-6.
[http://dx.doi.org/10.1016/S0531-5565(03)00167-0] [PMID: 14580875]

[2]   Leipzig RM, Sauvigné K, Granville LJ, *et al.* What is a geriatrician? American Geriatrics Society and Association of Directors of Geriatric Academic Programs end-of-training entrustable professional activities for geriatric medicine. J Am Geriatr Soc 2014; 62(5): 924-9.
[http://dx.doi.org/10.1111/jgs.12825] [PMID: 24749846]

## CHAPTER 2

# Health and Economic Consequences of Aging in US

**Rashmita Basu**[*]

*Texas A & M Health Science Center 8447 TX-47, Bryan, TX 77807, USA*

**Abstract:** The retirement of baby boomers and the rising share of elderly population are creating health and economic crises in the U.S. The U.S. Census Bureau projects that by 2030 there will be about 71 million Americans aged 65 and older and by 2040, one of every five Americans will be over 65 [1]. These demographics transitions have far-reaching implications for meeting healthcare needs and ensuring economic security for the elderly. As the Baby Boom generation ages, a large number of frail elderly will need health and personal care and progressively use more long-term care services which will have major implications for healthcare costs and public policies.

**Keywords:** Aging demographics, Baby boom generation, Demographics, Disability, Gender gap, Health care costs, Sociological change.

## INTRODUCTION

As individuals age, decline in functional status leads to an increasing need for personal care assistance with activities of daily living (ADLs) required to take care of oneself, such as bathing, toileting, eating, and dressing and instrumental activities of daily living (IADLs) such as cooking, grocery shopping, managing finances or medication. One recent study shows that after accounting for changes in sociocultural, economic and environmental factors between 1982 and 2009, successive cohorts of older adults are becoming more disabled over time [2]. It has been projected that by 2030 there will be over 21 million elderly limited in their activities and need assistance for a progressively long period of time.

In the U.S., the vast majority of personal care that allows older people to live in their communities is provided by family members as unpaid care. The combined effects of increasing older share of the population and greater life expectancy, the demand for long-term care services provided by unpaid caregivers will continue to increase. Due to private insurance policies in the U.S. professional caregiving is

---

[*] **Corresponding author Rashmita Basu:** Texas A & M Health Science Center 8447 TX-47, Bryan, TX 77807, USA; Tel: 254 721 1172; Fax: 254 724 4508; E-mail: Rashmita.Basu@bswhealth.org

not always provided. However, the traditional supply of unpaid caregivers is shrinking due to the gap between population growth rates of the elderly and people aged 25 to 54, particularly women who predominantly provide personal care. Beginning from 2025, the number of people aged 65 and over will exceed the number of women aged 25-54 (Fig. **1**). Due to increasing participation of women in the workforce (except long-term care workforce), marriage and reproductive trends (such as smaller family sizes) are restricting women's availability to care for family members. Outside of the U.S. these demographic changes are similar to many European countries. All these social and demographics changes will pose significant challenges to the elderly, policymakers, healthcare providers and planners to meet the care needs of older Americans and improve the lives of the family members who care for them.

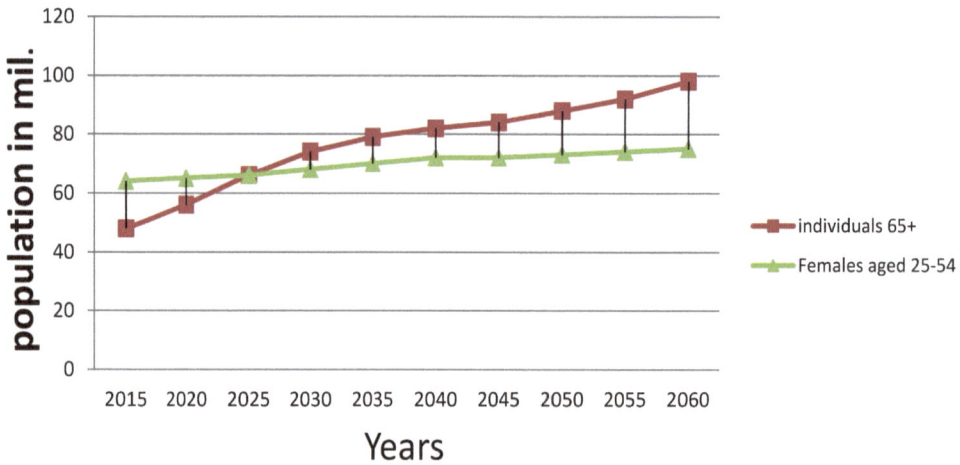

**Fig. (1).** Source: U.S. Census Bureau, Population Division, National Population Projections, Summary Files, "Total Population by Age and Sex, December, 2014.

The aging in general, and long-term care services in particular, will represent an overwhelming economic burden to the society and the healthcare system, including the public health system such as Medicare, Medicaid and other government sponsored programs. The other aspects of economic burden due to population aging include increase in Social Security payments, out-of-pocket medical care expenditures and cost for supplemental coverage for Medicare beneficiaries. The increasing number of people on Medicare and the aging of the Medicare population are expected to raise both the total and per capita Medicare spending. The current Medicare spending of $540 billion is expected to rise to $1 trillion by 2024. Since 2005, the rate of Medicare spending has been increased faster than the GDP in areas including skilled nursing facility (SNF), outpatient hospital, hospice, and lap services. This increased Medicare spending is contributed by the increase in Medicare population from 20 million in 1970 to 80 million in 2030.

The current study assesses the health and economic dimensions of the population aging in the U.S. The first part of this chapter discusses the logic that suggests the potential challenges for families and healthcare systems to meet the care needs of older Americans and the second part reviews the economic burden of aging in general and long-term care and Social security benefits in particular.

**Formal *versus* Informal Care**

In contrast to acute care, the vast majority (75%) of long-term care is unpaid or informal assistance provided by family and friends. As the older share of population is growing and people are living longer with chronic disabling conditions, particularly dementia, long-term care needs will become more challenging for families. Family caregivers are essentially the backbone of the delivery of long-term care needs of the elderly in the U.S. In general, adult children constitute the largest share of caregivers (42%) followed by spouse (25%), who provide assistance on personal care (*e.g.* bathing, toileting, dressing, and eating) and other instrumental activities (*e.g.* transportation for doctor appointment, bill payment, cooking, *etc.*). Although elderly who use informal care also use formal care (*e.g.* paid care from paraprofessional workers or nursing assistants) to supplement care needs. The following sections will focus on the availability and constraints of informal caregivers as long-term care is predominantly provided by the informal caregivers.

**Availability of Informal Caregivers and Constraints**

Informal caregivers of older adults are predominantly women. Informal caregivers and family caregivers are used to refer to individuals such as family members, partners, friends and adult child who provide care to older adults who have difficulty in performing activities of daily living in home and community setting. Estimates of number of informal caregivers in the U.S. vary depending on the definitions used for caregivers and care recipients as well as the types of care provided. For example, there are about 66 million informal and family caregivers who provide care to an elderly who is ill and disabled in the U.S. and about 27 million family caregivers provide personal assistance to adults with a disability or chronic illness [3]. Due to demographic transition and changes in socioeconomic circumstances, there will be a widening gap between care needs of the elderly and the availability of informal or family caregivers who can provide that care. This raises a concern for growing unmet care needs, a heavier burden on caregivers and increased demand for paid care. The combined effects of delayed childbearing, longer life expectancy, lesser proportion of middle-aged women who provide care contribute to unmet care needs and increased burden to the family caregivers. Furthermore, most of these middle-aged women in caregiving age are being "sandwiched' in their roles towards their children and aging parents. Wiemer and Beanchi [4] found that there was a 20% increase in the share of women who provide care to their children and aging parents between 1988 and 2007. Various other factors such as divorce, low fertility, and higher life expectancy will contribute to the fact that an increasing proportion of older adults aged 75 and over will have to live without an adult child or spouse [5].

## Dual Pressures of Informal Caregiving and Employment

*Caregiving in the U.S., 2015* highlights those workers with caregiving responsibilities for an adult with a disability or illness make up a substantial proportion of the labor force. About 60% of family caregivers caring for an adult also work for a paid job during their caregiving experience in 2014-an estimate of 24 million working caregivers of adults. These caregivers are more likely to be female (66%) than male (55%). About 63% of them were caring for an individuals aged 65 or older. In addition to their full-time job, on average, caregivers provide 34 hours per week on caregiving and many of them provide assistance to individuals with higher care needs. For example, about 28% of caregivers reported helping their care recipients with three or more activities of daily living (*e.g.* eating, bathing, dressing *etc.*) and more than half (about 54%) reported performing skilled nursing care (*e.g.* medication management). Caregivers in the age groups of 20 to 34 are more likely (73%) to engage in full-time (40 hours per week) employment compared to caregivers in any other age group which indicates that these young caregivers are facing the dual challenges of keeping their jobs and caregiving for an ill or aging family members. Although less prevalent, about 17% percent of caregivers are self-employed to better meet the care needs and work flexibility. Self-employed caregivers are more likely to be male, live with care recipients and report working fewer hours compared to caregivers work for an employer. The Employment pattern indicate that about 68% of Hispanic caregivers are in labor force compared with 60% of African American and 56% of White.

Providing uncompensated care for a family member while working full-time can be stressful. More than one-third of employed caregivers view that their caregiving situation is stressful emotionally and the lack of affordable supports services make it difficult to continue caring family members in the home or community setting. Balancing the dual responsibilities becomes particularly challenging for caregivers who lack the level of support services needed and unable to pay for the paid care. It is also common that caregivers need to adjust their work schedule (especially those involve in intensive caregiving) and take time off to meet the care needs of their care recipients. Furthermore, caregivers those who are employed full-time and could not afford to hire paid help, may have to leave the labor-force entirely and have to face financial stress due to loss of earnings and retirement benefits. Evidence suggests that higher-hours caregivers (*e.g.* providing 21 hours per week) are more likely (29%) to leave the labor market compared to caregivers (7%) who provide less than 20 hours per week. Some caregivers also report the experience of employment discrimination due to caregiving responsibilities. Typically caregiving for disabled elderly include assistance provided with limitations in activities of daily living (ADL) such as bathing, eating, dressing, toileting *etc.* and instrumental activities of daily living (IADLs) such as medication management, grocery shopping, cooking, transportation *etc.* (Table **1**).

**Table 1. Examples of Activities of Daily Living (ADL) and Instrumental Activities of Daily Living (IADL).**

| ADL | IADL |
| --- | --- |
| Dress | Cooking |
| Brush Teeth | Sweeping |
| Use Restroom | Buying Groceries |
| Bathing | Using Transportation |

## Caregiving With and Without Dementia

Caregiving experience is commonly perceived as a chronic stressor and caregivers most often experience negative psychological, behavioral and psychosocial effects which impact their quality of lives and general health [6]. For example, a recent study based on a nationally representative data, found that caregivers who provide care for 14 hours per week or more for more than two years are twice more likely to develop cardiovascular risk of cardiovascular disease compared to demographically matched adults who were not caregivers [7]. Another study found that becoming a caregiver can also increase the risk of developing depression among caregivers who provide care at least 14 hours per week or more. In 2013, about 40 million family caregivers provided 37 billion hours of care with an estimated value of $470 billion to their relatives, friends with chronic disabling conditions [3].

More than 75% of people with Alzheimer's disease related dementias (ADRD) receive care from family members and friends and they are considered as unpaid caregivers. In 2015, caregivers of people with ADRD provided about 18 billion hours of informal (*i.e.* unpaid) care which was estimated to be the value of $221 billion. The value of informal care was calculated as nearly as the costs of direct medical and long-term care of dementia in 2010 [8]. Although, the care provided to people with dementia is somewhat similar to the help provided to people with other chronic disabling conditions, caregivers of people with ADRD tend to provide more extensive care, possibly round-the-clock. Family caregivers with people with ADRD are more likely to monitor overall health of their care recipients and on average provide help with 2 ADLS and 5 IALDs compared to caregivers of people without ADRD (79% *versus* 66%). Based on the 2011 National Health and Aging Trends Study, caregivers of people with dementia are more likely to provide help with self-care and mobility (85% *versus* 71%) and medical care (63% *versus* 52%) compared to people without dementia, although about 50% of caregivers of people with ADRD report no experience of performing medical or nursing tasks. In addition to assisting with ADLs, caregivers of people with ADRD are more likely to manage finances, coordinate healthcare services and advocate for their care recipients with government agencies and service providers. Even after institutionalization to an assisted living facility or nursing home, some caregivers continue to provide assistance with ADLs.

## Economic Consequences of Aging

The two most important aspects of economic burden associated with population aging are: social security benefits and costs of financing long-term care and support services (LTSS). This section will review economic and financial challenges that the aging population will continue to face in the future years due to uncertainty of social security benefits and financing challenges for LTSS. Implications for public and private sectors on developing an effective long-term care support system for the elderly population and government policies on the long-term financial imbalances in the Social Security system are critical for ensuring economic well-being of the aging population in the future (Fig. **2**).

Expenditure for LTSS by Payer types, 2010

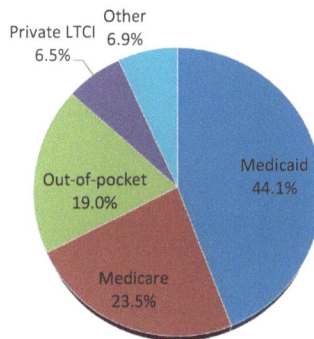

**Fig. (2).** Long-term care financing in the United States: Sources and Institutions [9].

## Economic Burden of LTSS

Expenditures for long-term care and support services (LTSS) represent a significant financial uncertainty for the elderly with approximately $320 billion in aggregate spending in 2011, or about 14% of all healthcare spending in the U.S. [10]. Going forward, long-term care expenditures are predicted to continue to increase due to combined effects of longer life expectancies and the numbers of "very old" who will disproportionately be the intensive users of LTSS [11]. For an individual after age 65, the present discounted value of expected LTSS cost was estimated about $50,000 with a 5% risk of incurring long-term care costs greater than $260,000 [12]. The majority of these costs are driven by nursing home care, where the average daily rate for a private room was $248 or $90,520 annually in 2012 [1, 13]. The financing of long-term care expenditure in the U.S. represents a significant challenge to the public sector as well as to consumers. Medicaid, the largest public payer, accounts for 44% of total long-term care expenditures [9], Medicare, the public health insurance benefits for older adults and disabled individuals accounts for about 23.4% of the LTC spending, but Medicare coverage for long-term care is limited in scope. Out-of-pocket spending for LTC comprises about 19% of total LTC expenses and private LTCI covers about 6.4% of LTC spending. However, it is important to recognize that families and friends provide a substantial portion of LTC because of limited coverage from publicly funded programs.

## Characteristics of LTCI Market

Long-term care insurance helps to pay for a variety of nursing, personal or support services for individuals who experience difficulties in performing daily activities due to chronic illnesses, disability or dementia. The services typically covered by LTCI range from assistance with activities of daily living (ADLs) such as bathing, dressing or eating as well as instrumental activities of daily living (IADLs) such as medication management, grocery shopping or preparing meals. This assistance is provided at home or in an institution such as assisted living facility or nursing home. A majority (approximately two-thirds) of active LTCI policies is purchased on an individual basis, while only a small percentage (less than one-third) of policies are purchased as group coverage through employer sponsored arrangement. All LTCI contracts are front loaded and the extent of front-loading varies across contracts. LTCI premiums are paid on a periodic (usually annually) basis at a pre-specified fixed rate determined at the time of purchase. In general, all LTCI policies are renewable and the premium is unaffected by any subsequent change in health condition or likelihood of the use of long-term care services in the future. While this means that premiums decline over time in real terms, the expected value of one year of coverage increases as health deteriorates. Therefore, premiums that individuals pay are initially higher than actuarial costs, but as their risk of using long-term care increases, the ratio of premium to risk falls [14]. However, insurers can and occasionally increase premiums for an entire "class of customers", especially if they discover that overall claims experience are higher than estimated earlier [15]. In 2010, individuals aged between 55 and 64 years who purchased a LTCI paid an average annual premium of $2300. This average policy includes a daily benefit of about $150 for four to five years, a 90-day elimination period, and a 5% inflation protection (AHIP 2012). Fig. (3) shows the future projection of LTC needs in the U.S.

Note: Annual costs for home health aide/homemaker services are based on 44 hours of care per week, multiplied by 52 weeks. Annual costs for adult day health care are based on a daily 6-8 hour rate for 5 days a week, multiplied by 52 weeks.

Majority of long-term care policies pay a fixed amount when the person needs care despite dramatic variability in the cost of services over time. These policies have a daily (or monthly) benefit amount and the policyholder will get reimbursed for the covered long-term care expenses that he/she incur up to this amount. Given the long-term nature of the contract, policyholders of LTCI typically continue to make payments for quite a long period of time before the risk of needing care becomes substantial. This means that although some of the long-term care risks are covered, but payments are made on an indemnity basis rather service basis (because of the intertemporal nature of the risk). Typical age for buying a private LTCI coverage decreased from 67 years in 2000 [16] to 59 years in 2010 (AHIP, 2012)-so on average, the policy is purchased substantially before the expected age of nursing home entry. For example, the average age of nursing home entry for a typical non-institutionalized 65 years old is 83 years [7], which is about 20 years after the average age of the policy purchase. Therefore, dropping a LTCI policy is costly to the insured as majority of policies do not have any surrender value and lapse of current policies always result in the forfeiture of any future benefits [11].

Median cost for selected LTSS in the US, 2012

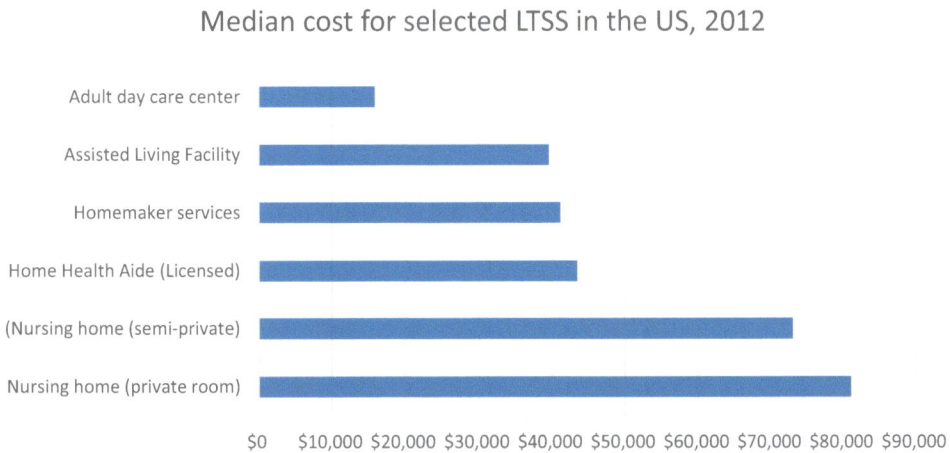

**Fig. (3).** Median cost for selected LTSS in the US, 2012. Source [13].

## Risks of using LTSS and Financial Challenges

As U.S. population aged 65 or older is projected to grow from 13% in 2010 to nearly 21% in 2050, the need for long-term care due to functional limitation will continue to increase. For example, individuals aged 65 or older, about 42% require assistance with performing daily activities (with ADLs or IADLs) due to functional limitations. The risk of experiencing disability increases from 6.5% in people between 65 and 69 to 43% among people aged 85 or older [15]. In particular, the likelihood of having 2 or more ADL limitations (usual criteria to qualify for Medicaid LTSS) increases by a factor of 6 when compares the 65 to 74 age group to that of 85 and older age group [1].

The pattern of functional limitation among older adults translates into the utilization of LTSS. The majority of individuals who require assistance for daily living in the community depend on informally provided help from friends and family. Although, recent statistics indicate the risk of using paid care among community-dwelling older adults ranges between 14 to 25% [17], the risk of using the nursing home care is significant. Based on the Congressional Budget Office estimate, 33% of individuals turning 65 in 2010 will likely to spend at least 3 months in a nursing home in their lifetime. However, the likelihood of using LTSS increases with age as well. For example, compared to 7.5% of individuals aged 65 to 74 use paid LTSS, about 31% of older adults over 85 years use paid care [15]. In the future years, the pattern of using paid care is likely to shift to the direction of greater use of paid LTSS as the ratio of adults aged 20 to 64 to those of 65 years of older will decline.

Life-time financial risks of needing LTSS for individuals from the age of 65 have been estimated in literature. For example, it is estimated the present discounted value of expected costs of LTSS for an individual turning 65 years of age is approximately $50,000, based on a simulation model [12]. Furthermore, authors claim that about 16% of those turning 65 would have lifetime costs of LTSS as $100,000 or more and about 5% would face a lifetime costs of $250,000 or more. However, a more recent estimate based on a simulation model of out-of-pocket healthcare spending shows that total lifetime healthcare costs for an individual turning 65 years of age would be $260,000, including expected costs of LTSS of $63,000. These numbers indicate that uninsured risks associated with LTSS may result negative impacts on consumption in retirement years. Recent literature also suggests that financing LTSS is one of the central reasons that drive older adults to declare bankruptcy [18].

Despite the size of economic burden of financing LTSS with limited publicly available resources, very little policy attention is given to designing private LTCI as an alternate approach to pay for LTSS. There are some financing options that have been proposed to consider: tax deductions for paying premiums of private LTCI, public provision of LTCI, and mandatory savings at younger age for self-insuring LTSS in the future. However, each of those has its own merits and drawbacks in order to be a viable financing option of meeting long-term care challenges in the future decades. Although, the tax deductibility for private LTCI premiums seem to boost the demand for private LTCI coverage, but the tax deductibility potentially could lower the after tax cost of insurance by 15 to 40% (range of marginal tax rate). Unfortunately, the largest share of benefits of this tax deductibility will be consumed by the wealthiest group of people, who most likely will not need to purchase private LTCI since they can self-insure themselves should they require LTSS in the future. Therefore, for the vast majority of the middle class people will not benefit much from the tax deductibility of the premiums with a 15 to 25% reduction in their premiums.

The most likely option for a public program for financing LTSS could involve a voluntary-type program financed by out-of-pocket payments for premiums similar to Medicare Part B. However, long-term sustainability of this type of program depends on various factors including financing mechanism and adverse selection problem. For example, The Affordable Care Act (ACA) of 2010 established the Community Living Assistance Services and Supports (CLASS) plan was designed as a voluntary publicly administered insurance program to help people should they need LTSS in any care settings such as home care, assisted living facility or nursing homes. The program is intended to pay people a fixed amount of cash benefits daily to pay for LTSS in return to premiums paid by them during healthy years. Therefore, this is self-sustaining program without any Federal supports and the current structure of the program does not appear to be financially viable or sustainable in the future years as acknowledged by many policy makers and administrators. Furthermore, it could be possible that people who know that they are high risk of using LTSS would be more likely to participate in the voluntary insurance program. This could impact the financial sustainability of the program because of limited premium dollars coming to the program compared to large payout in benefits coming out of the program. Therefore, so called "death-spiral" might occur with the possibility of increasing premiums which will discourage younger people from participating into the program.

The third type of financing option involves the mandatory savings in private investment accounts at young an age when annual savings become affordable. The annual savings will grow over the time period and when a person would turn 65 or higher, a private insurance option covering LTSS could be selected. However, this would mean that estimated savings rates should be enough for money to grow so that this financing mechanism would be viable. Furthermore, estimated savings will also depend upon market interest rate. Financing LTSS imposes significant financial challenge and economic burden on middle-class families. If some types of coverage-public, private or in combination will not become viable for paying LTSS, a significant portion of the aging population will face tremendous economic burdens of financing LTSS in the future decades.

**Economic Consequences of Aging: Social Security and Income Security after Retirement**

Social security is the foundation of retirement income for many older adults during retirement years in the U.S. In 2015, the Social Security system paid out $870 billion benefits to nearly 59 million beneficiaries and about 64% of beneficiaries received half of their income from Social Security in 2014 and about

66% of beneficiaries were retired workers [8]. Due to demographic transition and economic uncertainty, the system is currently facing a tremendous challenge of finding financial balance in the long run. Social Security benefits are projected to increase from 4.3% of gross domestic products (GDP) to 6.1% over the next 30 years while expected revenue is to be only 4.7% of GDP (Board of Trustees 2008). The challenge of financing retirement consumption of the elderly is not the only economic consequence of aging in the U.S., the Medicare and Social Security costs together are also projected to grow from 7% of GDP to 13% by 2035, imposing greater challenges for ensuring sustainability of Social Security finances for the future generations. Although it is evident that the reform in the Social Security system is essential, but the challenge is that demographic and economic factors that will determine the sustainability of Social Security finances are based on projections only. Therefore, any kind of reform in the Social Security system will involve either parametric changes (*e.g.* tax rates, benefit formula, eligibility age *etc.*) in basic financing mechanism of the system or fundamental changes in other personal financing program such as personal retirement accounts (PRAs). There are three types of changes that have been proposed for ensuring financial sustainability of the Social Security system in the future. The first proposed change is understanding uncertainty in demographic and economic forecasting and its implications for sustainable Social Security program. The second is the changes in the landscape of financial resources available to the retirees and their financial needs and resources have important implications for their retirement savings and therefore the Social Security benefits. Finally, understanding the influence of Social Security and other public policies on retirement decisions and delaying retirement that could potentially facilitate the economic transition of the Social Security system to accommodate demographic changes in older population group in the U.S.

## Uncertainty and Its Implications

Uncertainty regarding the financial solvency of the Social Security system is due to the projections of demographic and economic factors that are considered important for the finance of the system. A study quantifies the uncertainty in long-term projections of Social Security finances [12]. Based on a probabilistic model with various demographic variables (*e.g.* birth rates, death rates, growth of wage rates and the economy), authors proposed that at the median, payroll tax rate will need to increase by 5.1% to ensure sustainability in the Social Security system permanently.

Uncertainty in projection of mortality rates was addressed by Cutler, Glaeser and Rosen [18]. using data from National Health and Nutrition Examinations Survey (NHANES). The authors investigated impacts of health risk factors (such as smoking, drinking, obesity, and hypertension) and demographic factors (*e.g.* age, gender, race and education) on 10-year mortality rates and compared the predicted rates. The authors found that 10-year projected mortality rates decreased from 9.8% in 1971-1975 to 8.4% in 1999-2002. However, combined impact of fertility and mortality rates is uncertain and the divergence in fertility rates between different racial and ethnic groups as well as educational attainment is prominent and unless the source of this divergence is better understood, the uncertainty regarding fertility projection and its impact on Social Security finances will remain uncertain. Another uncertainty is the demographic changes attributed by the immigrants in U.S. Demographic characteristics (age distribution) and labor market activities (earnings, timing of retirement, Social Security tax) of immigrants have important implications for the solvency of the Social Security system. Comparing labor market behavior of immigrants to those of nonimmigrants, Borjas (2007) found the difference in employment rates between the two groups is dependent upon the "crossover" age which occurs in the late 50s or early 60s [16]. This is due to the eligibility requirements of receiving Social Security benefits in U.S. So, immigrants in their 50s who have not accumulated ten years of work in the U.S. would be reluctant to leave the job market because of earning the required employment credits for obtaining Social Security retirement benefits. This labor market behavior of nonimmigrants certainly impacts the Social Security liabilities. Although projection of these demographic and economic variables is important for formulating future trends but there is a great deal of uncertainty involved into this projection and hence the uncertainty about financial balance of Social Security system. This clearly indicates that we will need to have a reform in the Social Security system involving parametric changes that are more predictable and certain, for example, changes in the eligibility age, fixed change in benefits, fixed increase in payroll tax, or removing the earning cap for payroll tax rates.

## Financial Resources of Future Retirees

The landscape of financial resource needs and its availability to the future retirees has been changing with the increase in retirement savings in private sectors. However, increase in out-of-pocket medical care spending, along with demographic trends and changes in resource needs impact the financing of Social Security system. One of the most important trend affecting financial resources of future retirees is the transition from defined benefit retirement plans to defined contribution plans including 401(k) and other contribution plans. At present about 85% of private retirement savings programs include contribution from future retirees where individuals need to decide their contribution limits, investment allocation, and withdrawal time for ensuring the optimum return on their retirement income. Studies focused on transition to 401(k) and similar retirement plans found an increased participation in 401(k) retirement plans among those are eligible from 18% in 1984 to 34% in 1989 and 65% in 1999. Therefore, total equity assets in 401(k) retirement savings plans are projected to increase from $1.1 trillion in 2000 to $27 trillion in 2040 due to increased eligibility and participation rates in retirement plans. Although the projections are based on financial market performances but the trend in participation in defined contribution retirement plan would not change in the future. In addition to retirement savings, the accumulation of wealth in terms of housing equity has been changed over time. Due to recent volatility in the housing markets, new retirees have more housing equity and more mortgage debt than past retirees and possibility of changes in home value and home equity are also important component of the projection of housing wealth of the future retirees. Increased participation in 401(k) plans, plus Social Security income, together with lifetime earnings results a very dramatic shift in the landscape of financial resources available to the future retirees.

As the availability of financial resources has been changing over time, it is important to better understand factors that influence assets accumulation over time because impacts of these factors will determine if the transition to 401(k) retirement plans meet financial security of future retirees and any possible changes for improving these retirement savings plans. Specifically, there is a wide variation in 401(k) plans which may have different implications on savings behavior and retirement income. For example, a study led by Choi *et al.* [19] investigated impacts of plan level features such as automatic enrollment, employer's matching contribution, and default contribution rates on investment behavior related to 401(k) plans and founds that majority of people chose the default investment option rather than actively participating in choosing investment allocation in 401(k) plans. This may support the investment –based option in the Social Security system where the passive decision makers may choose default allocation in the private savings account for Social Security system. Furthermore, research has also shown that without employers' matching contributions in 401(k), the opt-out rate is relatively small which may indicate that automatic enrollment encourages individuals to participate in retirement savings plans. In addition to increased participation to retirement savings plans, the portfolio allocation decisions are important for financial protection of future retirees.

Studies have shown that number of different investment options (*e.g.* stocks, equities, bonds) impacts the way individuals make their asset allocation decisions and portfolio allocations may not always be in their best long-term interest. Therefore, selection of funds for retirement savings plans play an important role on how retirement savings will grow over time and meet financial needs of future retirees.

## Social Security, Health and Labor Market Behavior

Changes in health may impact one's ability to stay longer in labor market which in turn will have implications for Social Security finance. The prevalence of disability has declined in the last decade which implies that people can stay longer in the labor market which may reduce the financial challenges that the Social Security system is facing in the future. Healthier lives may lead to longer participation in labor market, increase in economic output and tax payment, and longer payment for social Security system. If Social Security incentives to leave the labor force at younger age can be removed and if health improvements can translate into grater physical capacity to stay in the labor force longer, then the proposed Social Security reform by increasing Social Security eligibility age may reduce the financial pressure on the system while maintaining the same benefit structure for future retirees. However, number of people receiving disability benefits has been increasing and therefore implications to the Social Security system is left for future research.

Retirement incentives inherent in the current Social Security system, optimum length of career in benefit calculations are some of the important factors that determine the retirement behavior. Social Security benefit calculation does not value the longer career beyond 35 years of age and thus benefit formula encourages career of 35 years or less [20]. The author also indicated that the benefit formula also disproportionately provides higher benefits to individuals with short career, treating them as same redistributive advantages as lower earning people.

The Social Security is currently experiencing about $13.1 trillion of unfunded liability and demand immediate reform for ensuring its financial solvency but increasing the payroll tax rate cap ($117,000) or eliminating the cap would not solve the financial shortfall of the system according to a recent study conducted by the Heritage Foundation. This will only increase the marginal tax rates for middle-income and upper-income wage earners and would be economically damaging. Increase in payroll tax could have negative impacts on the Social Security's financing challenges. Many economists confirm that any surplus in the

Social Security funds has not contributed to lower public debt rather increased government spending in other non-Social Security related areas. This is because surplus in Social Security fund is used in other government spending without having to borrow from external sources. Therefore, if the payroll tax cap increased then an influx of tax revenue in Social Security system will be used in non-Social Security spending and will not be "locked" in the Social Security fund for meeting future financial targets for older generation. Social Security reform is necessary for financial, but policymakers need to focus on reducing government spending and ensuring the original intent of the Social Security system *i.e.* prevention of poverty in old age. Increasing the payroll tax cap would likely to increase government spending in non-Social Security programs while reducing individual incomes, tax revenues and economic growth.

## Conclusion-Future Agenda

Challenges with log-term care financing and economic security of older adult demand immediate reform in social and public programs. One of the most important challenges related to aging population is maintaining healthy and productive aging. Healthy aging will increase disability-free years and lower the need for long-term care. At the same time keeping people healthy and productive could have significant economic impacts on financing long-term care costs and Social Security system for the future retirees. This is because, in addition to potentially lower demand for long-term care needs, healthier individuals are more likely to have greater physical capacity to work longer, require less long-term care supports and contribute to the Social Security system while delaying the retirement age.

The rate of disability in a population can be extremely variable and studies have shown that maintaining a healthy lifestyle (average level of physical activity) can potentially extend the onset of disability up to ten years with much lower lifetime disability. Currently, Americans spend 72% of their post 65 years of age with free of disability compared to 91% of the time among Japanese. Extending disability free time in older age will be equally significant compared to improving financing for long-term care. Advances in genomics and medicine along with better management of healthcare system (focusing on prevention rather treatment) could potentially lower the chronic disease and incidence of disability in older age. Extending disability free time in older age will potentially offer benefits to both financial challenges for long-term care system as well as Social Security system.

## CONFLICT OF INTEREST

The author confirms that author has no conflict of interest to declare for this publication.

## ACKNOWLEDGEMENTS

Declared none.

## REFERENCES

[1]    The State of Aging and Health in America 2013. http://www.cdc.gov/aing

[2]    Lin SF, Beck AN, Finch BK, Hummer RA, Master RK. Trends in U.S. Older adult disability: exploring age, period, and cohort effects. American J Public Health 2012; 102(11): 2157-63. [http://dx.doi.org/10.2105/AJPH.2011.300602]

[3]    Family caregiving in the U.S. Research Report; AARP Policy Institute, [last accessed Aug. 6, 2015]. http://www.caregiving.org/wpcontent/uploads/2015/05/2015_CaregivingintheUS_Final-Report-June-4_WEB.pdf

[4]    Wiemers EE, Bianchi SM. Competing demands from aging parents and adult children in two cohorts of American women. Popul Dev Rev 2015; 41(1): 127-46. [http://dx.doi.org/10.1111/j.1728-4457.2015.00029.x] [PMID: 26594071]

[5]    Ryan LH, Smith J, Antonucci TC, Jackson JS. Cohort differences in the availability of informal caregivers: are the Boomers at risk? Gerontologist 2012; 52(2): 177-88. [http://dx.doi.org/10.1093/geront/gnr142] [PMID: 22298747]

[6]    Schulz R, Sherwood PR. Physical and mental health effects of family caregiving. Am J Nurs 2008; 108(9) (Suppl.): 23-7. [http://dx.doi.org/10.1097/01.NAJ.0000336406.45248.4c] [PMID: 18797217]

[7]    Capistrant BD, Berkman LF, Glymour MM. Does duration of spousal caregiving affect risk of depression onset? Evidence from the Health and Retirement Study. Am J Geriatr Psychiatry 2014; 22(8): 766-70. [http://dx.doi.org/10.1016/j.jagp.2013.01.073] [PMID: 23791537]

[8]    2016 Alzheimer's disease facts and figures Alzheimer's & DementiaAHIP A guide to long-term care insurance 2016.

[9]    Frank RG. Long-term care financing in the united states: sources and institutions. Appl Econ Perspect Policy 2012; 34: 333-45. [http://dx.doi.org/10.1093/aepp/pps016]

[10]   Colello KJ, Mulvey J, Talaga S. Long-Term Services and Supports: Overview and Financing. Congressional Research Services; Working Paper. 2013; p. R42345.

[11]   Brown JR, Finkelstein A. Insuring Long-Term Care in the United States. J Econ Perspect 2011; 25: 119-42. [http://dx.doi.org/10.1257/jep.25.4.119]

[12]   Kemper P, Komisar HL, Alecxih L. Long-term care over an uncertain future: what can current retirees expect? Inquiry 2005-2006; 42(4): 335-50. [http://dx.doi.org/10.5034/inquiryjrnl_42.4.335] [PMID: 16568927]

[13]   The 2012 MetLife Survey of Nursing Home, Assisted Living, Adult Day Services, and Home Care Costs 2012. Access from https://www.metlife.com/assets/cao/mmi/publications/studies/2012/studies/mmi-2012-market-survey-long-term-care-costs.pdf

[14]   Finkelstein A, McGarry K, Sufi A. Dynamic Inefficiencies in Insurance Markets: Evidence from Long-Term Care Insurance. Am Econ Rev 2005; 95: 224-8.
[http://dx.doi.org/10.1257/000282805774669808]

[15]   Medicaid and Long-Term Care New Challenges, New Opportunities 2009. Accessed from http://www.lewin.com/content/dam/Lewin/Resources/Site_Sections/Publications/GenworthMedicaidandLTCFinalReport62310.pdf

[16]   Borjas G. Social Security eligibility and the labor supply of elderly immigrants RRC Paper No NB07-13. Cambridge, MA: National Bureau of Economic Research 2007.

[17]   Johnson RW, Wiener JM. A Profile of Frail Older Americans and Their Caregivers Retirement Project Occasional Paper 8. Washington, DC: The Urban Institute 2006.

[18]   Cutler DM, Glaeser EL, Rosen AB. RRC Paper No NB05-05. Cambridge, MA: National Bureau of Economic Research 2006; 1999-2002.Trends in risk factors in the United States, 1971-1975

[19]   Lindblad MR, Quercia RG, Riley SF, *et al.* Coping with Adversity: Personal Bankruptcy decisions of Lower Income Homeowners. Working Paper 2011.

[20]   Choi JJ, Laibson DL, Mardrian BC, Metrick A. Savings for retirement on the path of least resistance. In: McCaffrey EJ, Slemrod J, Eds. Behavioral Public Finance: Towards a New Agenda. Russell Sage Foundation 2006; pp. 304-52.

## CHAPTER 3

# Physical Changes in Age

**Daniela Fabiani-Longo, Kayla Bishop, James Mullen, Caitlin Murphy, Jesselee Allen, Virginia Cornelius, Jocelyn Dismore, Kathyrn McGeoch** and **Jeremy W. Grabbe**[*]

*The State University of New York, Plattsburgh, 101 Broad St. Plattsburgh, NY 12901, USA*

**Abstract:** There are a number of physical, psychological and social changes that occur with the passage of time. Aging, then, can be understood as the impact of time on our bodies. This happens on multiple levels, such as cellular and hormonal aging, accumulated damage, and metabolic aging. Well-being in late life depends on a tight-knit balance of physical, psychological, and social health [1]. If one of these three key components of a balanced life style is disrupted, it throws off the other two. For example, if an elderly individual suffers from flu, that in turn, will affect other aspects of their life. This individual may find it hard to be active when ill, which may lead to negative changes in their mood. In addition, other people may avoid him or her due to fear of catching their illness. This could lead to feelings of depression and social isolation, which may further impair immune system functioning.

**Keywords:** Balance, Cardiovascular changes, Hormones, Hypertension, Immune system, Osteopenia, Physical aging, Sarcopenia, Sensory changes.

## INTRODUCTION

Understanding how the major systems of the body are affected by aging can shed light on what changes are expected as a result of normal again and what change may be a sign of illness or disease. While people age at different rates depending on genetics, diet, culture, activity levels and environmental exposure, long-term population studies have given us clues about what changes we can expect. The focus of this chapter is to examine the physical changes that take place in the human body over time and how these changes impact the major systems of the body.

---

[*] **Corresponding author Jeremy W. Grabbe:** The State University of New York, Plattsburgh, 101 Broad St. Plattsburgh, NY 12901, USA; Tel: 1( 518) 792-5425; Email: jgrab001@plattsburgh.edu

## Muscular Skeletal System

The human body is made up of fat, lean tissue (muscles and organs), bones, and water. After age 30, people tend to lose lean tissue. Muscles, kidneys, the liver and other organs lose some of their cells. This process of muscle loss is called atrophy and as a result, this tissue loss reduces the amount of water in the body. Bones lose some of their minerals and become less dense (a condition called osteopenia in the early stages and osteoporosis in the later stages). The tendency to become shorter occurs among all races and both sexes. Height loss is related to aging changes in the bones, muscles, and joints. People typically lose about 1 cm every 10 years after age 40. Height loss is even more rapid after age 70. On average people lose a total of 1 to 3 inches in height as they age.. The main cause of the reduction in standing height is the loss of bone mineral content in the vertebrae, which leads to both collapse and compression in the length of the spine. Other causes of the reduction in standing height are changes in the joints and the flattening of the arches of the feet.

The weight loss that occurs in the later years of adulthood is not due to slimming of the torso but to the loss of lean body mass consisting of muscle and bone. Participation in exercise such as active sports can offset the effects of aging on body fat accumulation. Endurance athletes do not gain as much weight and they maintain their physical fitness for as long as they continue to train. Participation in exercise training programs can even be of value to adults who were more sedentary throughout their lives. By engaging in walking, jogging or cycling for about 3-4 days a week an individual can begin to see positive physical changes as soon as 10-20 weeks from starting the activity .

## Mobility

An individual's mobility is their ability to move around in their physical environment. This is a combined function of the integrity of the muscles, bones, joints, tendons, ligaments, and the contractibility of flexor and extensor muscles. Mobility changes throughout adulthood, to the extent that movement becomes more difficult, more painful, and less effective and efficient.

Between ages 40 and 70, there is a loss of muscle strength that amounts to approximately 10-20 percent. More severe losses occur between ages 70-80 (30-40%). However, there are individual differences that can lead to deviations from the general pattern of decline. The extent to which aging affects the loss of muscle strength depends upon gender, an individual's activity level throughout life, the particular muscle group tested, and whether the type of muscle strength tested is static or dynamic.

Bone development in adulthood is similar to muscle development in that it trends toward diminished skeletal strength. This results in a diminished ability of bones to withstand mechanical pressure, as well as showing a greater vulnerability to fracture. Decreases in various measures of skeletal strength range from 5-12 percent per decade starting in the 20s and continuing to the 90s. With time, microfissures develop in response to the stress placed on bones, which also contributes to the likelihood of a fracture.

Maximum skeletal strength loss ranges between ages 50 and 70. This is because the rate of reabsorption exceeds that of new bone growth in later adulthood. This results in the overall reduction of skeletal mass. Body weight is positively associated with bone mineral content, meaning that heavier individuals lose less bone mineral content and that less bone loss occurs in weight-bearing limbs. Genetic factors also play a role, as do lifestyle choices such as physical activity, smoking, alcohol consumption and diet. These factors can account for 50-60 percent of variance in bone density and also may influence the rate of fractures.

### Cardio-Vascular System

The most significant overall change regarding the cardiovascluar system in response to aging is reduced blood flow to the body, which typically becomes significant in the eighth decade. This results from a number of factors including normal atrophy of the heart muscle, especially in the left ventricle which pumps oxygenated blood out, calcification of the heart valves, loss of elasticity in artery walls (arteriosclerosis or "hardening of the arteries") and intra-artery deposits (atherosclerosis). The reduced blood flow results in reduced stamina since less oxygen is being exchanged, reduced kidney and liver function, and less cellular nourishment. As a consequence, the individual is more susceptible to drug toxicity, has a slower rate of healing, and a reduced response to stress. Other consequences of these cardio-vascular changes are hypertension with an increased risk of stroke, heart attack, and congestive heart failure [1].

### Respiratory System

As with the cardio-vascular system, there is also a reduction in the efficiency of the respiratory system in later life. The airways and lung tissue become less elastic with reduced cilia activity, resulting in decreased oxygen uptake and exchange. The muscles of the rib cage also atrophy, further reducing the ability to breathe deeply, cough, and expel carbon dioxide. These changes are exacerbated if the individual smokes or lives in a polluted environment. The consequences of these changes can include decreased stamina with shortness of breath and fatigue, which in turn may impair one's ability to perform activities of daily living. The lack of oxygen may also increase anxiety.

## Excretory System

Aging increases the risk of kidney and bladder problems including leakage or urinary incontinence (not being able to retain urine), urinary retention (not being able to completely empty the bladder), bladder and other urinary tract infections (UTIs), and chronic kidney disease [2]. With age, the amount of kidney tissue decreases, as does the number of nephrons, which are the cells that filter waste material from the blood. The blood vessels supplying the kidneys can become hardened and blood is filtered more slowly. In addition to changes in kidneys, the elastic tissue of the bladder's walls becomes tough and less stretchy over time resulting in a bladder that cannot hold as much urine as before. With age, the bladder muscles weaken, and the urethra can become blocked. In women, this can be due to weakened muscles that cause the bladder or vagina to fall out of position (prolapse). In men, the urethra can become blocked by an enlarged prostate gland.

Urinary incontinence is characterized by the complete or partial inability to control the urge to urinate. It is more common in women than men. The abnormality is usually caused by medications, weakness & abnormalities of bladder, bladder shrinkage and atrophy of urethra. However, incontinence can be successfully countered with bladder training, biofeedback, and the administration of anticholinergic drugs.

## Female Reproductive System

Aging changes in the female reproductive system result mainly from changing hormone levels. One clear sign of aging occurs when the menstrual periods stop permanently. This is known as menopause. The time before menopause is called perimenopause. It may begin several years before the last menstrual period. Some signs of perimenopause are: More frequent periods at first, and then occasional missed periods and periods that are longer or shorter. Along with changes in periods, physical changes in their reproductive tract occur as well. Menopause is a normal part of a woman's aging process. Most women experience menopause around age 50, though it can occur before that age. The usual age range is 45 to 55. With menopause, the ovaries stop making the hormones estrogen and progesterone, the ovaries also stop releasing eggs (ova). After menopause, women no longer become pregnant, menstrual periods stop. As hormone levels fall, other changes occur in the reproductive system, including: Vaginal walls become thinner, dryer, less elastic, and possibly irritated. Sometimes sex becomes painful due to these vaginal changes, Risk of vaginal yeast infections increases and the external genital tissue decreases and thins and can become irritated.

## Male Reproductive System

Everything that happens in the male reproductive system is part of changes in blood vessels and lack of elasticity of tissues among other things. Unlike women, men do not experience a major, rapid (over several months) change in fertility as they age (like menopause). Instead, changes occur gradually during a process that some people call andropause. Aging changes in the male reproductive system occur primarily in the testes, testicular tissue mass decreases. The level of the male sex hormone, testosterone stays the same or decreases gradually. There may be problems getting an erection. This is a general slowing, instead of a complete lack of function.

The tubes that carry sperm may become less elastic (a process called sclerosis). The testes continue to produce sperm, but the rate of sperm cell production slows. The epididymis, seminal vesicles, and prostate gland lose some of their surface cells. But they continue to produce the fluid that helps carry sperm. The prostate gland enlarges with age as some of the prostate tissue is replaced with a scar like tissue. This condition, called benign prostatic hypertrophy (BPH), affects about 50% of men. BPH may cause problems with slowed urination and ejaculation.

## Digestive System

Aging is a factor in several digestive system disorders. Older adults are more likely to develop diverticulosis (the presence of multiple balloon-like sacs (diverticula), usually in the large intestine), the strength of esophageal contractions and the tension in the upper esophageal sphincter decrease. The stomach lining's capacity to resist damage decreases, which in turn may increase the risk of peptic ulcer disease. The stomach cannot accommodate as much food (because of decreased elasticity), and the rate at which the stomach empties food into the small intestine decreases. However, these changes typically do not cause any noticeable symptoms. Aging has little effect on the secretion of stomach juices such as acid and pepsin, but conditions that decrease acid secretion, such as atrophic gastritis become more common [3].

Aging has only minor effects on the structure of the small intestine, so movement of contents through the small intestine and absorption of most nutrients do not change much. However, lactase levels decrease, leading to intolerance of dairy products by many older adults. Excessive growth of certain bacteria becomes more common with age, and can lead to pain, bloating, and weight loss. Bacterial overgrowth may also lead to decreased absorption of certain nutrients, such as vitamin B12, iron, and calcium, the pancreas decreases in overall weight, and some tissue is replaced by scarring (fibrosis).

## Autonomic Nervous System

A variety of functional and anatomical changes in the autonomic nervous system occur with age. These changes impair one's ability to "react" to environmental or internal stimuli that would normally be addressed with alterations in autonomic activity and a corresponding change in visceral functioning. The age-related functional declines of the visceral organs involve changes in receptor function and the loss of some autonomic projections. These end-organ changes cause, or are caused by, increases in activity in the sympathetic division of the autonomic nervous system, and possibly increases in activity in the parasympathetic division as well. Complicating matters further are critical changes in the balance and/or coordination of sympathetic and parasympathetic outflow to specific organs [4]. The basic question of what is actually the result of aging, an increased sympathetic (or parasympathetic) tone or a decreased responsiveness to sympathetic (or parasympathetic) activity, will be challenging to resolve because the two are so thoroughly intertwined. Declines in these autonomic nervous regulatory functions can significantly impair the quality of life of elderly patients.

## Sensory Systems

### *Visual System*

The decrease in quality of vision, particularly acuity, is the most noticeable with age. This often leads to poorer performance when engaging in daily tasks, greater sensitivity (not only to light, but also emotional sensitivity), inability of the eye to properly focus, and an overall reduction of visual acuity. As with other physical transformations of the body due to aging, the eye and surrounding area will undergo changes. When adults age, the eyelid muscles weaken; lids begin to droop, while the lower lid sags [5]. Eyelashes and eyebrows begin to thin out. Tear production reduces, decreasing the lubrication, often causing dry eyes or irritation. Conversely, opposite problems in drainage can lead to an excess of tears. As the build up leaks, adults experience watery eyes. When fat deposits build up, the white of the eyes may become a discolored yellow [5]. The color of the iris can change slightly as pigment cells begin to break down, causing some graying of the iris itself [6]. The retina becomes thinner due to reduction in the number of overall cells, also leading to a reduction in blood flow [5]. Pupils will also become smaller; a possible explanation is that this change makes it easier to focus when light goes through a smaller hole [6].

Normally, age-related changes occur not only on the entire eye as a whole, but also specifically on individual structures of the eye [7]. Beginning the fourth decade, the pupil begins to decrease in size and in response time to light. Because of these changes, it is estimated that older adults require three times the amount of illumination to see as a younger person. The lens of the eye becomes denser and opaque causing images to become dark or cloudy [1]. The retina will undergo change as the number of photoreceptors is reduced. The vitreous humor that fills the space between the lens and retina will begin to detach from the retina. "Senile meiosis" reduces the size of the pupil, resulting in less light reaching the eyes [8].

Along with quality of vision, the ability to focus on objects as they move closer or further away is impaired as people age. The fibers of the crystalline lens become harder and less elastic [9]. A buildup of yellow pigment in the lens (as well as possible debris) causes greater inability to discriminate colors, especially greens, blues, and violets [10]. The capability to see in low lighting becomes more difficult with age, for instance, in the case of night driving. Nyctalopia, or night blindness, is caused by damage to the light receptors (rods, but not cones) within the retina. Older adults have greater difficulty adjusting from bright light to dim light in general [1]. Scotomatic glare becomes a dangerous issue for aging adults when they are suddenly exposed to bright lights. The reaction time increases for an older adult to adjust from well-lit environments to darker environments. Driving at night becomes hazardous, not only because darker images are harder to perceive, but also quick flashes of high beams and/or glare from headlights can cause disorientation. This becomes especially dangerous for older adults when the changes in illumination are unexpected.

Perhaps the earliest sign of age-related vision changes is presbyopia, a form of farsightedness, where adults have difficulty seeing things close up. Older adults will begin holding reading material further from their face or eyes begin to feel strained and tired when trying to focus on fine print [5]. Interestingly, bright sunshine will reduce the impact of presbyopia. Also, those who were nearsighted in their youth may not experience the effects of presbyopia as severely [11].

Cataracts are the most common eye diseases from age-related changes. Roughly one half of Americans 75 and older can expect to develop a serious form of cataracts in their lifetime [11]. This clouding of the lens is caused by oxidation that damages the crystalline proteins of the lens. The intake of more antioxidants in our diet can reduce the risk of developing cataracts (Samuel).

Another common vision-related problem in older adults is glaucoma. Glaucoma is the second leading cause of blindness [11]. Cloud-angle glaucoma is caused by blockages in the eyes' drainage system, creating fluid back up that increases pressure on the optic nerve [5]. The outer edges of vision are affected first, and then a sort of tunneling effect into the center begins to occur [11]. Cloud-angle glaucoma affects peripheral vision and if left untreated, this condition can ultimately lead to permanent vision loss [5].

Age-related macular degeneration affects the part of the retina known as the macula, which is responsible for central vision. Older adults with age-related macular degeneration will have distorted vision of objects directly in front of them, in other words, a blind spot will appear directly in their line of vision [5].

Aside from serious, eye-related changes, older adults may experience visual phenomena that are not harmful, but simply cause annoyance. "Floaters" are spots that drift into our line of vision, caused by tiny groups of cells in the vitreous cavity [5]. The shadows of these clumps are cast onto the retina. They usually break apart without intervention, but sudden or persistent occurrence should result in consultation of a physician. "Flashes," also known as photopsia, are shooting-star-like flashes of light across the eye. They are caused by the vitreous gel pulling or rubbing against the retina.

As people age, they can take preventive measures or precautions to best limit the negative effects of age-related changes in vision or optimize their capacity under certain circumstances. In order to reduce the likelihood of eye problems or catch early signs of these problems, older adults should have routine eye exams or check-ups conducted by ophthalmologists, especially as they age [5]. Monitoring vision, taking proper vitamin supplements, and using protection against the sun (*i.e.* sunglasses) are all good preventative measures.

The risk of various vision-related problems increases even more so if a family history of varying vision issues is present. Age-related macular degeneration is the leading cause of blindness in older white adults. Older African American adults are affected most by cataracts and older Hispanic adults have the highest percentage rate of glaucoma [5].

### *Hearing*

Age-related hearing loss is known as presbycusis. Generally, both ears are affected by presbycusis. However, the delay between the onset of hearing problems and the time in which an individual actually seeks professional help to address the issue can be as long as 20 years [12]. Hearing changes that are common as we age include a decrease in sensitivity to high frequency tones and decreased discrimination of similar pitches. These changes are usually the result of normal changes to the bones and cochlear hair cells of the inner ear. Significant hearing loss, while relatively common in the elderly population, is not a normal part of the aging process. Approximately 30% of all elderly persons have some hearing impairment. Such loss is usually the result of damage to the hearing organ, the peripheral nervous system, and/or the central nervous system. Depending upon the specific cause and location of the problem, different types of hearing loss may result, including high tone loss, flat hearing loss, and difficulty understanding or distinguishing words. The most common form of hearing loss is reduced sensitivity to high frequency tones. Men are more susceptible to this form of hearing loss than women. In addition, as people age it becomes difficult for them to hear when there is interference or distractions. Tinnitus (ringing in the ears) is another issue that can occur as we age. It consists of abnormal ear noise that can be caused by wax build up or medicines that may damage structures within the ear. Because hearing deficits make it hard for older people to hear noises present in their immediate environment, hearing loss leads to both impaired physical functioning as well as psychological difficulties. For example, feelings of social isolation or loneliness might result from not being able to hear, and as a consequence engage in, conversations with family members or friends. Failing to hear doctor's recommendations, fire alarms or sirens could also jeopardize an individual's physical health.

Most hearing changes are not amenable to medical or surgical intervention, hearing aids and aural rehabilitation are usually indicated, although not all types of hearing loss are remediable. Interventions that teach how to decode the facial patterns associated with individual sounds (bottom-up training) and how to use contextual cues embedded in speech (top-down training can be successful as well [12]. Because hearing is essential for social interaction and safety, untreated hearing loss is perhaps the most socially disabling of all sensory impairments. It is an invisible disability which is often covered up or denied by a person who may then be mislabeled as senile, demented, or uncooperative.

### *Gustation and Olfaction*

Taste and olfaction are grouped together as "chemical senses." There is a general decrease in people's taste sensitivity and a concomitant decrease in the ability for them to detect odors. These changes can impact the quality of one's life (missing out on pleasurable aspects of food) and may also pose a threat to safety and well-being (such as failing to detect the smell of a gas leak or spoiled food). The loss of taste may lead to improper diet and contribute to, or accelerate certain aspects of aging. With age there is a reduction in the total number of taste buds, especially after age 80. As a consequence of these changes include a decreased interest in food, a desire for more salty or highly seasoned food, and a reduced awareness of body odor and environmental hazards such as spoiled food, smoke, and hazardous fumes.

### Tactile Perception

With advanced age, the skin becomes somewhat less sensitive to sensation, including heat, cold, and injury. While this is relatively inconsequential for most people, it can pose a serious threat for those whose insensitivity is extreme. Perhaps more important, however, is the recognition that touch is one of our most important senses all through life. It serves many important functions such as forming a sense of self, relieving stress, giving comfort, maintaining intimacy, and conveying acceptance and connectedness. Because older adults typically have less opportunity to give and receive touch, they may lose the benefits that these functions impart.

Temperature perception is another factor that changes as adults age. Once an individual reaches age 65 they become impaired in their responses to hot and cold temperatures. This in return can increase the risk of injury from frostbite, hyperthermia, and burns. As humans age, the ability for them to be able to raise their core temperature, when the body's peripheral temperature becomes diminished. Due to the decreased secretion of sweat glands in the skin, elder people, experience impaired responses to extreme heat. Most aging adults are less likely to drink water under conditions of heat stress due to reduced thirst sensitivity. Reduced sensation of thirst in older people is associated with a tendency to lose water with urine. Their kidney's age along as they age and the ability to respond to sodium load is impaired. This can lead to cellular volume expansion and hypertension. On the other hand because an aging body is less adaptable to outside temperatures, adults living in colder areas may restrict their outdoor activities.

## Endocrine System

### *Immune System*

The immune system is a complicated network of cells, tissues, and organs to keep us healthy and fight off disease and infection. The immune system is composed of two major parts: the innate immune system and the adaptive immune system. Both change as people get older. Our ability to survive the germs around us is based on a tightly controlled immune system. Too little of an immune response makes us susceptible to infection, including life-threatening pneumonia. Conversely, an overactive immune response is at the root of autoimmune diseases common among older people and may contribute to age-related chronic diseases like Alzheimer's disease, osteoarthritis, diabetes, and heart disease [13]. Given the delicate balance of the immune system, gerontologists suspect that, along with its more obvious negative consequences, immunosenescence (the gradual deterioration of the immune system brought on by natural age advancement), might have a protective role in older adults.

The immune system is our body's primary defense against bacterial, viral, and parasitic infections, as well as their toxic byproducts, and abnormal cells such as precancerous and tumor cells. The innate immune system consists of cells and proteins that are always present and ready to mobilize and fight microbes at the site of infection. The main components of the innate immune system are: 1) physical epithelial barriers, 2) phagocytic leukocytes, 3) dendritic cells, 4) a special type of lymphocyte called a natural killer (NK) cell, and 5) circulating plasma proteins. The adaptive immune system, on the other hand, is called into action against pathogens that are able to evade or overcome innate immune defenses. Components of the adaptive immune system are normally silent; however, when activated, these components "adapt" to the presence of infectious agents by activating, proliferating, and creating potent mechanisms for neutralizing or eliminating the microbes. There are two types of adaptive immune responses: humoral immunity, mediated by antibodies produced by B lymphocytes, and cell-mediated immunity, mediated by T lymphocytes [13].

As we age our immune systems change. As a result, elderly individuals do not respond to immune challenges as robustly as the young [14]. Autopsy studies have revealed that the thymus gland, which produces T cells that are designed to fight new strains of bacteria and viruses starts to deteriorate shortly after sexual maturity is reached. There is some evidence that the remaining T cells are able to produce an enhanced response despite their smaller numbers. One of the most recognized consequences of aging is a decline in immune functioning. While elderly individuals are by no means immunodeficient, they often do not respond effectively to novel or previously encountered antigens. The effects of aging on the immune system are manifested at multiple levels that include reduced production of B and T cells in bone marrow and thymus and diminished function of mature lymphocytes in secondary lymphoid tissues [1].

Researchers have explored ways of optimizing the immune system. The relationship between exercise and immune function is complex. Most researchers agree that to decrease the risk from immune system aging it is important that as you age you get plenty of exercise, eat healthy, do not smoke, get the vaccines your health care provider recommends, and look into safety measures to prevent falls and injuries. Researchers have also examined affective states such as stress and depression, nervous system functioning and the immune system. The results were interesting. For example, elderly individuals with high levels of stress experience lower T cell functioning which means that they are more likely to become ill. Conversely, social support, at least in women, was found to be positively related to immune system competence measured in terms of lymphocyte numbers and response to mitogens [1]. So, in contrast, individuals with healthy social outlets, experience lower levels of stress which may actually lead to a healthier immune system. The environment that the individual is exposed to can also have an enormous effect on their immune system functioning. In the studies on mice, researchers found considerable variation in the aging of their immune systems. This applied even between mice who were housed together. A factor in immune system health could be the social order of the participant mice. Whether the mice are in a submissive or dominant social position, it could result in stress that in turn could affect patterns of gene expression causing immune variations [15].

This environmental stress also applies to humans. Current research has shown that life stress in humans can decrease the activity of telomerase, the enzyme that is responsible for maintaining the protective sequences of DNA at the end of chromosomes, suggesting that social and environmental influences can impact the aging process [15].

## CONCLUSION

This chapter has revealed how age affects the major physical systems in the body. However, physical aging is not a process in which the entire body begins to change in unison; each system of the body changes at its own pace and the rate of these changes depends upon the individual's biology, environment and lifestyle.

## CONFLICT OF INTEREST

The authors confirm that they have no conflict of interest to declare for this publication.

## ACKNOWLEDGEMENTS

Declared none.

## REFERENCES

[1]     Cavanaugh JC, Whitbourne SK. Gerontology: an interdisciplinary perspective. New York, NY: Oxford University Press, Inc. 1999.
         [http://dx.doi.org/10.1093/med:psych/9780195115468.001.0001]

[2]     Testa A. Understanding urinary incontinence in adults. Urol Nurs 2015; 35(2): 82-6.
         [PMID: 26197626]

[3]     Fillit HM, Rockwood K, Young J, Brocklehurst JC. Brocklehurst's textbook of geriatric medicine and gerontology. 7th ed., Philadelphia: Saunders 2010.

[4]     Hotta H, Uchida S. Aging of the autonomic nervous system and possible improvements in autonomic activity using somatic afferent stimulation. Geriatr Gerontol Int 2010; 10 (Suppl. 1): S127-36.
         [http://dx.doi.org/10.1111/j.1447-0594.2010.00592.x] [PMID: 20590828]

[5]     Fine LC, Heier JS, Corliss J. The aging eye: Preventing and treating eye disease. Boston, MA: Harvard Health Publications 2012.

[6]     Anshel J. Healthy eyes better vision: Everyday eye care for the whole family. Los Angeles, CA: The Body Press 1990.

[7]     Scheie HG, Albert DM. Textbook of ophthalmology. 9th ed., Philadelphia: Saunders 1977.

[8]     Carter JH. Predictable visual responses to increasing age. J Am Optom Assoc 1982; 53(1): 31-6.
         [PMID: 7056988]

[9]     Cook CA, Koretz JF, Pfahnl A, Hyun J, Kaufman PL. Aging of the human crystalline lens and anterior segment. Vision Res 1994; 34(22): 2945-54.
         [http://dx.doi.org/10.1016/0042-6989(94)90266-6] [PMID: 7975328]

[10]   Mancil GL, Owsley C. Vision through my aging eyes revisited. J Am Optom Assoc 1988; 59(4 Pt 1): 288-94.
         [PMID: 3397476]

[11]   Samuel MA. Macular degeneration: A complete guide for patients and their families. Laguna Beach, CA: Basic Health Publications 2008.

[12]   Pichora-Fuller MK, Levitt H. Speech comprehension training and auditory and cognitive processing in older adults. Am J Audiol 2012; 21(2): 351-7.
         [http://dx.doi.org/10.1044/1059-0889(2012/12-0025)] [PMID: 23233521]

[13]   Chandra RK. Nutrition and the immune system: an introduction. Am J Clin Nutr 1997; 66(2): 460S-3S.
         [PMID: 9250133]

[14]   Montecino-Rodrigue E, Berent-Maoz B, Dorshkind K. Causes, consequences, and reversal of immune system aging. J Clin Invest 2013; 123(3): 958-65.
         [http://dx.doi.org/10.1172/JCI64096] [PMID: 23454758]

[15]    Dorshkind K, Montecino-Rodriguez E, Signer RA. The ageing immune system: is it ever too old to become young again? Nat Rev Immunol 2009; 9(1): 57-62.
[http://dx.doi.org/10.1038/nri2471] [PMID: 19104499]

## CHAPTER 4

# Cognitive Changes in Aging

**Ann McCarthy**[1] and **Jeremy W. Grabbe**[2,*]

[1] *John Carroll University, 1 John Carroll Blvd, University Heights, OH 44118, USA*

[2] *The State University of New York, Plattsburgh, 101 Broad St. Plattsburgh, NY 12901, USA*

**Abstract:** As people get older, they begin to worry that any type of memory lapse may be the onset of dementia. In fact, the American Psychology Association agrees that dementia is one of the most feared aspects of getting older. It may be important, therefore, for both aging individuals and potential caretakers to have a better understanding of what would be considered to be normal age-related cognitive changes and what would be considered to be changes that might indicate a condition that would need to be evaluated by a medical professional.

**Keywords:** Attention, Cognitive changes, Dementia, Long-term memory, Memory, Methodology, Mild cognitive impairment, Short-term memory.

## INTRODUCTION

What if you encountered a woman wandering through a parking lot looking for her car? Would you be worried that she had dementia or would you assume that she just forgot where she parked? Likely, your answer would depend on the woman's age. We often attribute memory lapses in younger people to be the result of stress, not paying attention, or some other relatively harmless reason, yet for the same memory error in an older person, most of us, including older adults, would attribute the cause to possible dementia or delirium. For the record, I never have been able to remember where I park my car. This includes my adolescent years, my younger adult years, and my middle age years. I'm not expecting the situation to improve in the next twenty years! I am sure, however, that the reaction of people around me will change as they begin to attribute the exact same behavior that has been present for many years to age-related changes rather than to an issue that I've had my entire life.

* **Corresponding author Jeremy W. Grabbe:** The State University of New York, Plattsburgh, 101 Broad St. Plattsburgh, NY 12901, USA; Tel: 1( 518) 792-5425; Email: jgrab001@plattsburgh.edu

**Jeremy W. Grabbe (Ed.)**

So, do cognitive declines or changes occur as people get older? This would be a short chapter if this were an easy question to answer! The "common sense" answer is that of course it is normal to experience cognitive changes as one ages. The scientific answer is much more complicated because cognition itself is complex. The answer to the question is both "yes" and "not so much", or "quite a bit", depending on the aspect of cognition being examined. It may also depend largely on the research design used to assess potential cognitive differences between younger and older adulthood.

The answers to these questions are important not just from a human development perspective, but they also have an impact on everyday living situations. Do cognitive changes/declines occur at a particular age so that society may need to apply a maximum age allowed for driving an automobile? Is it acceptable to raise the age to receive social security because not only are people living longer but they are also certainly capable of remaining in the job force? Should there be a mandatory retirement age for some professions due to inevitable cognitive declines? These are not easily answered questions, and it might behoove us, as a society, to consider the actual research rather than our "common sense".

One of the concepts to understand before discussing the most commonly used research designs is the difference between age-related changes and age-related differences. Age-related change means that whatever is different between an older person and a younger person is due strictly to getting older. For example, a common age-related change that occurs is presbyopia, which is a form of far-sightedness. As people get older, normal changes in the eyes (such as thickening and hardening of the lens, less flexibility of the lens) cause them to not be able to see things that are close as well as they did when they were younger. Again, these physical changes are commonly due to aging. Age-related differences are simply things that are different between two or more cohorts of individuals. For example, younger people do not see a problem with an unmarried couple cohabitating before marriage, whereas a person in his seventies might be quite distressed that his granddaughter is "living in sin". There is a clear difference in moral thinking, but this cannot be attributed to getting older. The gentleman in his seventies was probably not more inclined to think that this was acceptable when he was in his twenties, either. Unfortunately, many times research results are often interpreted as being age-related changes rather than age-related differences.

Another common misinterpretation of research findings involves correlations. Correlations are statistics that are used to describe variables and relationships between variables. One cannot assume, however, that one variable CAUSES a change in another variable. A common example is that ice cream sales increase when the temperature increases. By the same measure, ice cream sales decrease when the temperature decreases. Suppose two variables behave in the same manner, both increasing and both decreasing. This is a positive correlation. When variables move in opposite directions, one increasing as the other decreases, this is known as a negative correlation. For example, as a student spends increasing time playing video games, her grade point average will decrease. It is important to note that we just cannot conclude that one variable is causing the other reaction. We just do not know what other things might contribute to the relationship. For example, it makes sense that because it is hot outside that people eat more ice cream in an attempt to decrease body temperature. Another reason for the positive correlation may be that more people are going to more places that offer ice cream as a food choice – like fairs, carnivals, zoos, amusement parks, *etc*. We simply do not know because we have not accounted for those types of variables. So, we cannot conclude that warmer weather itself causes people to eat more ice cream, and we certainly cannot reach the conclusion that if we all agree to eat more ice cream, it will cause temperature to increase! We can, however, predict that as it gets hotter outside, ice cream sales will increase.

These types of statistics are often misreported in the media and come to be accepted by the general public. For example, there is a correlation between solving crossword puzzles and/or other mentally stimulating cognitive tasks and dementia [1, 2]. These researchers found that older people who regularly solve crossword puzzles (or partake in other cognitive activities) often have much lower rates of dementia than older people who are not solving crossword puzzles. This is a negative correlation (more puzzles = less dementia). This information CAN be used to PREDICT the incidence of dementia (Mr. Jones does not solve crossword puzzles and may be more likely to suffer from dementia), but it cannot be said that doing crossword puzzles CAUSES people to avoid dementia. Yet, in the media, correlations are quite often presented as causing certain events to occur or not occur. Unfortunately, most people are not reading professional journals or books and take this information as it presented in the media.

A common misconception about most aging research is that these are true experiments, but in reality, there are no studies on age comparisons that can be considered true experiments. (In fact, both of the previously mentioned studies regarding crossword puzzles rely on self-reports of cognitively demanding activities and none of the groups were measured at a baseline and then performed tasks and were later measured). In order to be considered a true experiment, the researchers must have randomly assigned each participant to a condition. This means that each participant had an equal chance of being assigned to a particular condition. It is not possible to randomly assign a participant to the "older adult" or "younger adult" group, nor is it possible to randomly assign a participant to a "dementia" or "non-dementia" group. An experiment should also have included random sampling. This means that in the general population, each individual had an equal chance of being chosen to participate in the experiment. Younger adults are recruited from college campuses. Younger adults in the general population may not be truly comparable to college students. A true experiment should also include an independent variable – the variable that we are hoping will have an effect or change on the results of the experiment, and a dependent variable – the way that we are measuring our results. Lastly, there should also be an experimental group of participants who have randomly been assigned to receive the treatment or manipulation (the independent variable), and a control group that does not receive the treatment or manipulation. By including a randomly assigned control group, it can be more strongly concluded that whatever differences that are found between the experimental and control group can be attributed to the independent variable.

Again, when examining most age comparison research, these are not true experiments, and therefore it is inappropriate in most cases to conclude that any particular variable caused a change. Participants cannot be randomly assigned to the age variable, they are most probably not selected from the general population, and there cannot be a control group that receives none of the manipulation, one of which is of course age itself. You simply do not have a control group that does not age as another comparison group. Therefore, most aging studies are considered to be quasi-experiments. Aging research usually cannot fulfill all of the requirements to be considered a true experiment. That is not to say that valuable information regarding age changes and differences cannot be inferred through this type of research, but rather one needs to be careful about how the data is interpreted.

## AGING AND CONGNITIVE CHANGES

Taking all of these factors into consideration, there are some age-related cognitive changes that are considered "normal" and are not indicative of dementia, delirium, or other abnormal mental defect. Three of the most important factors to consider are attention, memory, and intelligence.

## ATTENTION

Attention is essential for most cognitive tasks. If you aren't paying attention in class, you probably will not be learning (encoding). If you are not paying attention while you are driving, you have just increased the odds that you will be involved in a traffic accident. Many of our everyday missteps can probably be attributed to lack of attention. Although we all think that we understand what we mean by the term "attention", attention is like most cognitive concepts, more complex than what is seems.

There is not really a definition of attention on which all professionals can agree. Some general ideas about attention include the notion that attention requires some type of mental resources. These resources are limited, and there is only so much in our environments on which we are able to focus our attention. Our attention is also quite flexible, and we can often choose where we focus our attention.

It might be more beneficial to look at attention through the goal that is trying to be accomplished. Four types of attention include executive attention, sustained attention, selective attention, and divided attention.

Executive attention is our ability to direct, manage, and control our attentional resources in order to successfully complete a task. This type of attention affects decision-making, judgments, emotional responses, and planning, as well as other demands such as language comprehension, reading, and social behavior. Driving a car is often used as an example to illustrate executive attention because of the great number of competing demands involved in this activity. Executive attention involves more than simply focusing on demands, however. Another important element is the ability to inhibit (or ignore) stimuli in the environment that are irrelevant to the task. Studies involving cell phone use while driving often rely on measuring executive attention. Executive attention is also rather limited. We can only pay attention to only so much information at one time, and when we are bombarded by too many stimuli, we simply ignore some incoming information. Executive attention is negatively affected by age. Mahoney, Verghese, Goldin, Lipton, and Holtzer [3] used the Attention Network Test (ANT) to assess healthy older adults' executive attention abilities. In this measure, a target arrow pointing left or right is cued by information on each side of the target (flankers). These flankers can be congruent, incongruent, or neutral with the target. The participant is also cued as to spatial location of the flankers before the target appears. These researchers found that as age increased, executive functioning ability decreased, particularly the ability to resolve the issue of the conflicting flankers.

Sustained attention is when someone is trying to stay focused on a particular stimulus. When you're sitting at a traffic light and waiting for it to change to green, you are likely watching the light so that you can begin moving as soon as it switches. This is sustained attention. Of course, there are many different occurrences that can interrupt your sustained attention to the light. Someone might dart in front of your car, there may be a loud noise, or someone attractive may drive up next to you. It takes quite a bit of mental resources to control sustained attention, especially when a task is not particularly difficult or engaging. Research results regarding age-related changes in sustained attention have been mixed. McDowd and Shaw [4] conclude age-related changes in sustained attention are few and minimal but older adults may experience more detriment when target location is uncertain and when targets appear more frequently [5].

Selective attention is the process by which a person chooses on what they will be paying attention. Selective attention is thought of as a controlled process because people do have a choice about where their attention is focused, although selective attention may require more mental resources at some times rather than at others. Some factors that may affect selective attention are level of fatigue, how intriguing the task, current emotional state, the amount of information to be processed. One of the most important features of selective attention is the ability to ignore or inhibit irrelevant information. The conclusion of many studies is that older adults find it much more difficult to inhibit responses to irrelevant information and therefore they may experience more difficulty when attempting to focus attention and disregard other stimuli [4].

Divided attention means that you have to pay attention to more than one stimulus or more than one task at the same time. In popular terms, you have probably heard the term "multi-tasking". Usually, both tasks are somewhat equal in importance, but people being what they are, often unconsciously "choose" one task over the other. This is one of the main reasons that it is so dangerous to talk on a cell phone when you are driving. If you are an experienced driver, you probably feel like driving is something that you have much expertise doing, so it is alright for you to talk on the phone as that is not a particularly difficult task either. When push comes to shove, however, that phone conversation is probably much more interesting than the road, which does not seem to change all that much. When the car in front of you suddenly stops, however, it is easy to belatedly comprehend that divided attention while driving is not effective. In the lab, divided attention is measured by performance using a dual task paradigm. Participants often perform two tasks separately, and then are asked to perform both tasks simultaneously. Any increased reaction time and/or decreased accuracy when both tasks are performed simultaneously is considered to measure a cost of multi-tasking. Rogers and Fisk [6] suggest that although it is commonly assumed that older adults have a higher cost in divided attention tasks compared to younger adults, older adult performance may be influenced by complexity of the task, how often the task has been practiced, and whether the elements of the tasks in and of themselves are measuring an age-related decline. Another consideration is the motivation of the participants. Older adults generally have difficulty with locomotion than younger adults, and older adults also generally suffer more consequences if they fall. When given the dual task of memorizing items using the method of loci and concurrently walking on a treadmill, older adults were more likely to abandon the memory task to better focus on the walking task, whereas the opposite was true for the younger adults [7]. Older adults were also more likely to utilize a handrail as an aid for walking as the task demands increased, whereas the younger adults were more likely to use an aid for the memory task.

Two of the most important factors that affect attention (and memory, which will be discussed in the next section) are speed of processing and processing resources. Speed of processing refers to how quickly one is able to process environmental stimuli early in the attentional process. For example, when waiting for a traffic light to change to green, how quickly does someone recognize that it has changed to green and how quickly does she respond to that change? Processing resources is a bit more vague term. When psychologists speak of processing resources, they are referring to the amount of mental energy required to allocate attention to a stimulus or task. If a task has become automatic, the task requires few processing resources. For adults, tying a shoe requires few attentional resources, and adults can do many other tasks while tying that shoe. To a young child, however, many processing resources are necessary to complete the task. He may need to focus on the shoe strings, may have to talk himself through the steps, try more than once to complete the task, and he really cannot focus on much else than tying the shoe. In fact, if you try to speak to him while he is tying his shoe, he might become very frustrated because you have overloaded his attentional capacity.

## MEMORY

In television, movies, and books, memory is often portrayed to be akin to a photograph or video. The event is available in long-term memory, in the exact form that the event took place. It is important to consider, however, that these fictional accounts do not really reflect what memory is and what function it serves. Memory is a subjective reconstruction of an event. In other words, not only does the event become part of the memory trace, all of the emotions, previous experiences, and personal bias also play a role in what is remembered. By using this definition, it is easy to understand how two people remember the same event quite differently.

We'll be looking at different aspects of memory for this chapter. We'll consider immediate memory, explicit/implicit memory, long term memory, and retrospective and prospective memory.

## INFORMATION PROCESSING MODELS

To put it simply, when we talk about cognition in terms of information processing, we are simply drawing an analogy between how a computer works and how the human mind works. We have information coming in (encoding), we find a place to keep it (storage), and later we need to get that information back out (retrieval). As a computer comparison, you type your paper on your computer (encoding), hit the "save" button frequently (storage), and then later you simply double click the file to retrieve it.

One of the most widely known information processing models is the Atkinson-Shiffrin or modal model [8]. The first stage in this model involves sensory memory. Sensory memory is an extremely brief form of memory that is based on either visual stimulation (iconic memory) or auditory stimulation (echoic memory), or any of the other senses. Sensory memory fades rather quickly, but for a short amount of time, a brief memory trace can be expected and a "memory" of the sensory event is retained [9]. Currently, this phenomenon is often referred to as neurological persistence. The next step in the modal model is short-term memory. This is a temporary store for information that may or may not be converted to long-term memory. If the to-be-remembered information is not repeated or rehearsed, it is forgotten. This information is available on a very limited time basis (estimates vary from 15 to 20 seconds) and also has a very limited capacity estimated five to nine items could be held in short term memory [10]. The last step in the process is long-term memory. This is the long-term store for general information, autobiographical memory, and procedural memories. Long-term memory is believed to have unlimited capacity.

Previously, it has been believed that age-related changes in sensory memory are minimal. More recent research, however, has demonstrated that auditory sensory memory declines with age [11]. Furthermore, Cooper, Todd, McGill, and Michie [12] found that older adults may require longer auditory processing times than younger adults, thus leading to auditory sensory memory declines. Recent evidence also suggests that visual sensory memory may also require longer processing time for healthy older adults and may also indicate mild cognitive impairment if this decline is especially evident [13].

# IMMEDIATE MEMMORY

Immediate memory is usually conceptualized as the type of memory required to keep items in mind for a fairly short time. For example, if you need to remember a few items at the grocery store or a phone number until you can find a pen to write it down, you would be utilizing what many professionals would consider to be short-term memory. When using short-term memory, most people simply repeat the to-be-remembered information until the task has been completed. According to Craik [14], there seem to be very few age-related changes in short term memory, and when age differences have been found, the differences although significant, are often quite small.

Another aspect of immediate memory is working memory [15]. Although it can be argued that short-term memory is necessary for working memory, working memory is a much more complex concept. The Baddeley and Hitch model suggests that working memory is composed of a master system (the central executive) and two separate subsystems (the phonological loop and the visuospatial sketchpad). The central executive is responsible for allocating memory resources, task-switching, controlling attention, inhibition of irrelevant information/stimuli, and language, and reasoning. The phonological loop is responsible for processing verbal stimuli, and the visuospatial sketchpad is responsible for processing visual and spatial stimuli. The most significant difference between short term memory and working memory is the manipulation of the to-be-remembered information. If I need to remember five specific items at the grocery store and keep repeating those five items to myself, I am using short term memory. If I am trying to remember what I need based on a recipe that I hope to use for dinner that evening, I not only have to remember specific items, but I may also need to go through the steps to complete the meal, the order that I would add the ingredients, and any "extra" items like oil for frying or salt for seasoning. In other words, I am not only repeating information to myself but also manipulating that information while holding the previous steps in memory. This would largely be processed by the phonological loop. If I am imagining the groceries necessary to complete my shopping, then I am probably using the visuospatial sketchpad. Unfortunately, the age-related declines in working memory are well-documented [14]. Older adults appear to be able to retain the ability to hold information for a limited time in short term memory, but then they experience difficulty when required to manipulate information or when the task becomes more complex [14]. Although these findings are robust, other research has indicated that declines may be more specific for visuospatial tasks rather than phonological [16].

## IMPLICIT AND EXPLICIT MEMORY

Another aspect of memory to consider is the difference between actively trying to remember information for later recall or recognition (explicit memory) or unconsciously remembering information that we can recall or recognize later even though we never actively processed that information for later recall or recognition (implicit memory). Explicit memory is often measured by tests with which we are all familiar – essay tests, recognition tests (*e.g.* multiple choice tests), *etc*. Implicit memory is often measured by priming tasks, word completion tasks, and word stem tasks. Implicit memory also includes procedural memory – memory of how to do things. Tying your shoe, riding a bike, or ice skating are examples of procedural memory.

The research regarding implicit memory is optimistic. There seems to be very few and/or very small age-related changes in implicit memory. In fact, Fleischman [17] believes that any deficits in implicit memory may be an indicator of disease or mental cognitive impairment. In her meta-analysis, she contends that implicit memory differences between younger and older adults is often confounded by research design (longitudinal studies show little decline compared to cross-sectional studies), undiagnosed cognitive impairment effects, small sample size, and tasks that do not measure implicit memory that are not confounded by explicit memory.

The evidence for explicit memory is not quite as optimistic, but is also not always so clear cut so that we can say that there are definitive age-related declines in explicit memory. The testing method itself can demonstrate both declines and maintenance. Older adults typically perform much worse than younger adults when utilizing recall. Recall tasks involve much more deliberate cognition and higher processing skills. In an early study, Schonfield and Robertson [18] found that although younger adults outperformed older adults on recall, there was no significant difference on the recognition task. More recently, Danckert and Craik [19] also demonstrated these effects, and they also provided evidence that frontal lobe and hippocampal function declines could be related to the decline in recall memory.

## LONG-TERM MEMORY

Another way to examine memory is to consider long-term as opposed to immediate memory. Like most psychological concepts, there is disagreement as to this distinction. For simplicity, consider that long-term memory is the long duration storage of all learned material that may be limitless. It includes knowledge of yourself and all the information that you have learned throughout your lifetime. Long-term memory is typically divided into nondeclarative memory and declarative memory. Nondeclarative memory is sometimes used interchangeably with the concept of implicit memory in that it typically includes procedural memory, conditioning, motor memory, and unconscious learning. Because of the similarity of these concepts, we can assume that like implicit memory, there are few age-related declines in nondeclarative memory, and when age differences are found, these differences are typically small even if significant.

Declarative memory is further divided into episodic and semantic memory. Semantic memory is thought of as general knowledge and facts that someone has about the world. It typically includes all the things that you learn in school, work-related knowledge and expertise. There are usually very few emotional components involved in the recall of semantic memories. For example, you may remember that the capitol of Ohio is Columbus, but you cannot specifically remember where you learned that fact nor does that fact make you feel elated or depressed. Episodic memory is more subjective than semantic memory. Episodic memory includes the "episodes" of your life, whether that event happened days ago, years ago, or just a few minutes ago in a laboratory setting. Most laboratory research about long-term memory is based on episodic memory.

It is important to remember that there is not necessarily always a clear division between semantic and episodic memory. For example, I do know that Columbus is the capitol of Ohio (semantic memory) AND I remember that I learned that fact in Mr. Schwallie's seventh grade Ohio history class (episodic memory). Mr. Schwallie was one of my favorite teachers, so there is a small positive affective component to that memory (episodic memory), which is usually triggered by going places in Ohio and the history about the state that I learned in that particular class (semantic memory). Many times, however, we know information or facts (semantic memory) but have little memory from which we learned the fact, when we learned it, or how we learned it.

Age-related deficits for semantic memory are typically small, and based on longitudinal studies; often do not occur until very late in life. Ronnlund, Nyberg, Bäckman, and Nilsson [20] conducted a five year longitudinal study and found that semantic memory may increase until about the age of sixty. They also suggested that educational attainment effects may be a critical variable to consider when researching both semantic and episodic memory. Many times even cross-sectional research finds few declines in semantic memory. For example, Nyberg *et al.* [21]. conducted an extensive cross-sectional study on semantic, episodic, and implicit memory effects, and as expected, found few age differences in semantic memory ability and priming, but they found significant age differences in episodic memory. Age-related deficits in episodic memory are well-documented, and older adults have particular difficulty in recall tasks.

## RETROSPECTIVE *VS.* PROSPECTIVE MEMORY

Another difference in how we can look at memory is retrospective memory and prospective memory. So far, everything that has been covered has been about retrospective memory – things we remember from past experiences. Immediate memory, long-term memory, autobiographical memory, and explicit/implicit memory are all types of memory of things from the past. On the other hand, prospective memory involves remembering to do something in the future. For example, successfully remembering a dentist appointment, remembering to take a medication, remembering to pick up your child from school, remembering to complete a homework assignment, all involve the accuracy of your prospective memory.

Prospective memory is akin to "remembering to remember" something, so it is like having to remember something twice. You not only have to remember to do this future task, but you need to trigger some other stimulus about it. It would seem that this "double" processing should show an age-related decline, but the results are mixed. There are actually two types of "triggers" for prospective memory, event-based triggers and time-based triggers. An example of an important function would be taking medication compliance, and this might be especially important to older adults who typically take more medications than other age groups. If Joe needs to take his medication with a meal, before bedtime, or upon waking in the morning, he would be using event-based triggers to trigger his prospective memory to take his medication. Event-based triggers happen when something external to a person, such as meals and waking, occur to remind that person to perform a particular action. If, however, he needs to take his medication at a specific time (*e.g.* 10:00 am) or in specific time increments (*e.g.* every four hours), he must rely more heavily on internal cognitive cues to remember to take his medication. (It is possible to change an event-based trigger into a time-based trigger by adding an external cue, such as an alarm, when it is time to take the medication).

Azzpardo, Jehel, and Auffray [22] conducted a study not only examining event-based and time-based prospective memory, but they also considered the different results that may be obtained in a laboratory setting *versus* a naturalistic setting. Studying only older adults, their findings indicate that older adults were able to complete laboratory tasks in both event and time-based prospective memory, although event-based performance was significantly better than time-based. These researchers also found that the participants performed well on the naturalistic setting in both types of prospective memory tasks. Interestingly, they found that retrospective memory skill and processing speed and more importantly, executive flexibility (being able to shift tasks) were also quite influential in success in prospective memory tasks.

Therefore, in the world outside of the laboratory, however, healthy older adults are usually more effective at remembering appointments, taking medications, *etc.* than younger adults. This difference between the laboratory findings and real-life settings might be explained by how salient (important) these activities are to the performers. For example, it could be that it is more important to an older person to arrive and to arrive on time for appointments than it may be for a younger person. Due to this difference in social cognition (what we think or know about appropriate social behavior), an older adult may be more likely to use external aids, such as alarms and calendars, than would a younger adult. By doing so, the older adults are compensating for prospective memory losses in a way that makes performance much more similar to that of a younger adult.

## INTELLIGENCE AND WISDOM

If an alien were to watch television as an attempt to discover the effects of age on intelligence, she might come to the conclusion that the most intelligent representatives of our species are about eight to twenty years of age, with adolescents being at the peak of intellect. Television has a tendency to portray this age group as the cleverest, wittiest, and most knowledgeable about everything. In particular, this younger age group is especially intelligent about the "real world", as they are the only ones who usually know what is going on in their worlds. Middle-age persons, if they are shown at all, are usually parents who can only hope that their clever children will be able to help the family cope with disasters and problems. Lastly, older adults are usually shown to be completely inept with any type of technology, have no clue about what is going on in the world or even right in front of them, and it seems like they should be in a nursing home. Because of the popular portrayal of aging individuals in this country, many people assume that there is an inevitable age-related loss of intelligence.

## INTELLIGENCE

Professionals simply cannot agree on a definition of "intelligence", but many can agree on some basic characteristics of intelligence. Intelligence is generally believed to be comprised of the ability to adapt to situations, to acquire knowledge (not necessarily school knowledge), problem-solving and reasoning ability [22]. Although school performance may not be the only way to measure intelligence, these characteristics do often predict an individual's school performance.

There simply is not enough room in this chapter to discuss each and every intelligence measure and theory and potential age-related differences and changes. We can, however, look at some basic elements of intelligence and examine some general trends regarding age and intelligence.

## FLUID *VS.* CRYSTALLIZED INTELLIGENCE

Cattell & Horn conceived the notion of intelligence into being two separate abilities. Crystallized intelligence is what would be exhibited in school-type behaviors, such as language skills and the acquisition of general knowledge. Crystallized intelligence is often measured by vocabulary tests and general knowledge tests, or can be used in trivia or word games. Fluid intelligence is the ability to solve new or novel problems, to be able to solve problems that require insight or being able to see all possible consequences of a decision or answer, to reach conclusions from multiple sources of information, to recognize patterns or relationships among stimuli, and abstract problem solving. Fluid abilities are often measured by letter or number series completion tasks, the Ravens Matrices measure, and puzzles such as Sudoku.

It is generally accepted that age has different effects on each of these forms of intelligence, and the research is quite robust in the findings. Fluid abilities reach a peak in the mid-twenties, and then begin a gradual decrease throughout the lifespan whereas crystallized intelligence increases until very late in life. Through the use of Sudoku puzzles, Grabbe [23] found a correlation between working memory and the ability to successfully complete the puzzles which suggests that there is a correlation between working memory and fluid intelligence. It has also been suggested that fluid intelligence is driven by more biological factors, such as speed of processing and neuronal activity. Bugg *et al.* [24] found that processing speed and frontal lobe functioning were also significant factors in the ability to perform fluid abilities tasks. Crystallized intelligence seems to be driven more by environmental factors such as level of education and continued intellectual development activities. Interestingly, Ghisletta, Rabbitt, Lunn, and Lindenberger [25] suggest that fluid intelligence and crystallized intelligence may not be quite as disconnected as previously believed. These researchers studied participants from early old age to later old age, and they found that crystallized intelligence declines were correlated not only with fluid intelligence loss but also with lifestyle factors, disease, and impending death.

Paul Baltes proposed a different way of looking at intelligence. He also considered intelligence as two different types – the mechanics and the pragmatics of intelligence. The mechanics of intelligence is heavily reliant on the physiological condition of the brain and is exhibited in tasks that involve speed of processing, perceptual speed, and reasoning ability. The pragmatics of intelligence are more reliant on cultural factors, such as school performance or practical problem solving. You could also say that fluid intelligence is somewhat like the mechanics of intelligence because both are biologically based and that crystallized intelligence is somewhat like the pragmatics of intelligence since culture is an important component of both. In fact, the trajectory for the mechanics and pragmatics of intelligence follows a very similar path to their counterparts. Mechanics peak in the mid-twenties and then follow a slow steady decline across the lifespan, whereas pragmatics gradually increase throughout the lifespan, reaching a peak in midlife and not noticeably decreasing until very late in life [26].

It has also been suggested that expertise may mitigate some of the declines in fluid intelligence. Experts are people who have a great deal of experience and practice with a specific skill that has accumulated over a significant amount of time. For example, Charness [27] found that chess experts are often able to maintain or even improve their standing until very late in life. Yet they experience the same slower processing speed of other older adults. Their repeated practice with this specific skill seems to allow them to compensate for slower processing speed perhaps by knowing strategic short-cuts, more plausible moves by an opponent, *etc.* Unfortunately, this compensatory mechanism is only viable for the specific skill. For example, an expert chess player will take the same amount of time to learn a new game as would a non-chess-playing older adult.

As much of the time intelligence is measured by standardized tests (a.k.a. psychometrics), it should always be kept in mind that there are often very large individual differences in not only overall scores but also the specific area of intelligence being measured. It is possible that Mary has a greater overall decline than Theresa, but Theresa experienced greater losses in math than in verbal ability and she may in fact score higher than Mary in verbal ability. Another factor to keep in mind that is that health may play an important role in the score of an intelligence measure. Many of the subtests that may tap into fluid intelligence are timed tests. In other words, if an individual has not yet completed the task in the allotted time, it is considered "incorrect". Some of these types of tasks include manipulating small blocks or small cards. If someone has arthritis, these seemingly simple tasks can be painful and slow. Vision and hearing changes may also affect scores. If an older adult cannot properly hear directions (and they may be reluctant to ask for clarification), performance will suffer. If the writing on the testing materials is too small or difficult for them to see, performance may suffer. If lighting is insufficient, performance will suffer. If utilizing a computer, researchers and practitioners also need to be aware of lighting conditions as well as the level of glare when administering a measure to an older adult. Many older adults also have not had the same educational opportunities compared to many younger adults, and may not have attended school for the same amount of time. Older adults have often been out of school much longer than their younger counterparts and are no longer used to taking tests, sitting still for extended periods of time, and encountering the type of problems often on these tests.

Some factors may affect both younger and older adults when taking these tests as well, but may affect older adults more so. For example, if anyone is fatigued, his/her performance on an intelligence measure will suffer. An older adults' performance may suffer more than a younger adult's, especially if the older adult is tested in the afternoon or evening. Anderson, Campbell, Amer, Grady, and Hasher [28] found that older adults' peak intellectual performance occurs in the morning and declines as late afternoon approaches. Using *f*MRI, these researchers also found that in the morning, older adults' scans were more similar to younger adults' scans, particularly in the middle frontal gyri and parietal regions. Finally, it is been suggested that if anyone goes into a testing situation and is anxious about performance due to some personal characteristic, such as race, gender or age, being tied into a stereotyped belief about themselves based on this characteristic, performance may suffer. This is known as stereotype threat, and some research does suggest than when individuals hold beliefs that they will perform less well on a test, this negative attitude can have a negative impact on test scores. Chasteen, Bhattacharyya, Horhota, Tam, and Hasher [29] induced stereotype threat in older adults, and then gave the participants several memory tasks. Results indicated that performance on both recall and recognition tasks suffered as a result.

## WISDOM AND EVERYDAY INTELLIGENCE/SOCIAL COGNITION

Other researchers have suggested that once people are through with education; most no longer have need of the same skill set in order to be successful. The notion of "everyday" intelligence is similar to what is referred to as "common sense". What should you do if your babysitter cancels and you need to go to work? What should you do if a hamburger catches on fire on your stove? Nancy Denney suggested that the answers to these types of questions are more important to determining intellectual functioning than are traditional intelligence measures. One method of study was to give different age- specific vignettes to different age groups. Denney expected that each age group would perform best on their problem, Most of her research, however, found a steady increase in the ability to solve these types of everyday problems through middle adulthood, and then people experienced a slow but steady decrease in successful solutions [30]. In other words, the middle-aged adults performed best on all age-specific vignettes.

Another way of looking at lifelong intelligence might be labeled wisdom. Wisdom is the lifelong accumulation and practical application of knowledge, especially about social issues, behavior, and problems. Perhaps older people, who presumably have vast experience in dealing with the world, have acquired an expertise on handling various dimensions of social activities and problems. Paul Baltes felt that the other measures of intelligence lack this aspect of social expertise and attempted to demonstrate that older adults' wisdom has been underestimated and undervalued. In a series of experiments [31], presented younger, middle-aged, and older adults were presented with everyday problems and social dilemmas specific to their age group, and then evaluated the level of wisdom exhibited when solving the problems. The results of the initial experiments were comparable to those found by Denney – middle-aged adults exhibited more wisdom in their responses then the other two age groups. On a positive note, older adults did perform a bit better on "their" questions as compared to the other age-specific question, but middle-aged adults still performed best on all of the questions. Smith and Baltes [31] also noted, however, that not many of the research participants in ANY age group responded with "wise" answers. They concluded that not many people are wise, but if you exhibit wisdom when you are younger, this is not a skill that you will lose later in life [31].

## NORMAL *VS.* ABNORMAL COGNITIVE LOSS

All of the presented information has been about normal cognitive changes related to aging. Many older adults often begin to fear Alzheimer's disease or other dementias as soon as they forget where they put their glasses or wallets, or forget to send a birthday card, or have other minor memory lapses. People in every age group can be forgetful, so how can we know when attentional, memory, or intellectual declines are something that need to be more fully examined? The first indicator that a cognitive loss can no longer be considered to be a part of normal aging is the performance of activities of daily living (ADLs). ADLs include tasks such as dressing oneself, feeding oneself, bathing, toileting, and walking. When an individual begins to repeatedly struggle with these very basic self-care activities, a medical exam is probably warranted. Instrumental activities of daily living (IADLs) are more complex activities that are also required for independent living to be successfully accomplished, and difficulty in performing these types of activities may in fact be one of the first indicators that an older adult may no longer be able to care for him/herself. IADLs include activities like paying bills on time and managing money and budget, household maintenance, doing laundry, shopping, transportation or arranging transportation in the event that an individual does not drive, taking medications appropriately, and planning and preparing meals. Deficits in these activities may also indicate that cognitive declines have reached a degree when a person is no longer safe when taking care of himself/herself [32].

Another factor to consider is the degree to which the cognitive decline affects the quality of daily living. An older adult who begins to show difficulty with IADLs who also has an adult child who lives nearby can live at home much longer than an older adult without such a support system. However, when ADLs, which are much more personal, such as toileting and feeding oneself, a relative or close friend who lives nearby may no longer desire (or even be able) to assist with care any longer.

## CONCLUSION

In conclusion, it can sometimes be frightening and confusing when cognitive impairment may be a serious condition to consider as one ages. Individuals, spouses, and caretakers are affected by abnormal declines and the responsibilities and loss that they may incur as a result of impairment. Even when decline is considered normal, precautions should be taken to ensure safe and positive environments to lead to successful and healthy aging.

## CONFLICT OF INTEREST

The authors confirm that they have no conflict of interest to declare for this publication.

## ACKNOWLEDGEMENTS

Declared none.

# REFERENCES

[1]     Pillai JA, Hall CB, Dickson DW, Buschke H, Lipton RB, Verghese J. Association of crossword puzzle participation with memory decline in persons who develop dementia. J Int Neuropsychol Soc 2011; 17(6): 1006-13.
        [http://dx.doi.org/10.1017/S1355617711001111] [PMID: 22040899]

[2]     Landau SM, Marks SM, Mormino EC, *et al.* Association of lifetime cognitive engagement and low β-amyloid deposition. Arch Neurol 2012; 69(5): 623-9.
        [http://dx.doi.org/10.1001/archneurol.2011.2748] [PMID: 22271235]

[3]     Mahoney JR, Verghese J, Goldin Y, Lipton R, Holtzer R. Alerting, orienting, and executive attention in older adults. J Int Neuropsychol Soc 2010; 16(5): 877-89.
        [http://dx.doi.org/10.1017/S1355617710000767] [PMID: 20663241]

[4]     McDowd JM, Filion DL. Aging, selective attention, and inhibitory processes: A psychophysiological approach. Psychology and Aging 1992; 7: 65-71.
        [http://dx.doi.org/10.1037/0882-7974.7.1.65]

[5]     Mouloua M, Parasuraman R. Aging and cognitive vigilance: effects of spatial uncertainty and event rate. Exp Aging Res 1995; 21(1): 17-32.
        [http://dx.doi.org/10.1080/03610739508254265] [PMID: 7744168]

[6]     Rogers WA, Fisk AD. Understanding the role of attention in cognitive aging research. In: Birren JE, Schaie KW, Eds. Handbook of the psychology of aging. San Diego, California: Academic Press 2001; pp. 267-87.

[7]     Li KZ, Lindenberger U, Freund AM, Baltes PB. Walking while memorizing: age-related differences in compensatory behavior. Psychol Sci 2001; 12(3): 230-7.
        [http://dx.doi.org/10.1111/1467-9280.00341] [PMID: 11437306]

[8]     Atkinson RC, Shiffrin RM. Human memory: A proposed system and its control processes. 1968.
        [http://dx.doi.org/10.1016/S0079-7421(08)60422-3]

[9]     Sperling G. A model for visual memory tasks. Hum Factors 1963; 5: 19-31.
        [PMID: 13990068]

[10]    Miller GA. The magical number seven plus or minus two: some limits on our capacity for processing information. Psychol Rev 1956; 63(2): 81-97.
        [http://dx.doi.org/10.1037/h0043158] [PMID: 13310704]

[11]    Cheng CH, Lin YY. The effects of aging on lifetime of auditory sensory memory in humans. Biol Psychol 2012; 89(2): 306-12.
        [http://dx.doi.org/10.1016/j.biopsycho.2011.11.003] [PMID: 22120681]

[12]    Cooper RJ, Todd J, McGill K, Michie PT. Auditory sensory memory and the aging brain: A mismatch negativity study. Neurobiol Aging 2006; 27(5): 752-62.
        [http://dx.doi.org/10.1016/j.neurobiolaging.2005.03.012] [PMID: 15908049]

[13]    Lu ZL, Neuse J, Madigan S, Dosher BA. Fast decay of iconic memory in observers with mild cognitive impairments. Proc Natl Acad Sci USA 2005; 102(5): 1797-802.
        [http://dx.doi.org/10.1073/pnas.0408402102] [PMID: 15665101]

[14]    Craik FI. Age-related changes in human memory. In: Park DC, Schwarz N, Eds. Cognitive aging: A primer. Philadelphia, PA: Psychology Press 2002; pp. 75-92.

[15]    Baddeley AD, Hitch GJ. Working memory. In: Bower GH, Ed. The psychology of learning and motivation. London: Academic Press 1974; Vol. 8.

[16] Oosterman JM, Morel S, Meijer L, Buvens C, Kessels RP, Postma A. Differential age effects on spatial and visual working memory. Int J Aging Hum Dev 2011; 73(3): 195-208. [http://dx.doi.org/10.2190/AG.73.3.a] [PMID: 22272505]

[17] Fleischman DA. Repetition priming in aging and Alzheimers disease: an integrative review and future directions. Cortex 2007; 43(7): 889-97. [http://dx.doi.org/10.1016/S0010-9452(08)70688-9] [PMID: 17941347]

[18] Schonfield D, Robertson BA. Memory storage and aging. Can J Psychol 1966; 20(2): 228-36. [http://dx.doi.org/10.1037/h0082941] [PMID: 5942327]

[19] Danckert SL, Craik FIM. Does aging affect recall more than recognition memory? Psychology and Aging 2013; 28: 902-9. [http://dx.doi.org/10.1037/a0033263]

[20] Ronnlund M, Nyberg L, Bäckman L, Nilsson LG. Stability, growth, and decline in adult life span development of declarative memory: Cross-sectional and longitudinal data from a population-based study. Psychology and Aging 2005; 20: 3-18.

[21] Nyberg L, Bäckman L, Erngrund K, Olofsson U, Nilsson LG. Age differences in episodic memory, semantic memory, and priming: relationships to demographic, intellectual, and biological factors. J Gerontol B Psychol Sci Soc Sci 1996; 51(4): 234-40. [http://dx.doi.org/10.1093/geronb/51B.4.P234] [PMID: 8673644]

[22] Snyderman M, Rothman S. Survey of expert opinion on intelligence and aptitude testing. Am Psychol 1987; 42: 137-44. [http://dx.doi.org/10.1037/0003-066X.42.2.137]

[23] Grabbe JW. Sudoku and working memory performance for older adults. Act Adaptation Aging 2011; 35: 241-54. [http://dx.doi.org/10.1080/01924788.2011.596748]

[24] Anderson JAE, Campbell KL, Amer T, Grady CL, Hasher L. Timing is everything: Age differences in the cognition control network are modulated by time of day. Psychology and Aging 2014; 29: 648-57. [http://dx.doi.org/org/10.1037/a0037243]

[25] Ghisletta P, Rabbit P, Lunn M, Lindenberger U. Two thirds of the age-based changes in fluid and crystallized intelligence, perceptual speed, and memory in adulthood are shared. Intelligence 2012; 40: 260-8. [http://dx.doi.org/10.1016/j.intell.2012.02.008]

[26] Baltes PB. The aging mind: potential and limits. Gerontologist 1993; 33(5): 580-94. [http://dx.doi.org/10.1093/geront/33.5.580] [PMID: 8225002]

[27] Charness N. Search in chess: Age and skill differences. J Exp Psychol Hum Percept Perform 1981; 7: 467-76. [http://dx.doi.org/10.1037/0096-1523.7.2.467]

[29] Chasteen AL, Bhattacharyya S, Horhota M, Tam R, Hasher L. How feelings of stereotype threat influence older adults memory performance. Exp Aging Res 2005; 31(3): 235-60. [http://dx.doi.org/10.1080/03610730590948177] [PMID: 16036721]

[30] Denney NW, Pearce KA. A developmental study of practical problem solving in adults. Psychol Aging 1989; 4(4): 438-42. [http://dx.doi.org/10.1037/0882-7974.4.4.438] [PMID: 2619950]

[31] Smith J, Baltes PB. Wisdom-related knowledge: Age/cohort differences in response to life-planning problems. Dev Psychol 1990; 26: 494-505. [doi]. [http://dx.doi.org/10.1037/0012-1649.26.3.494]

[32]    Lawton MP, Brody EM. Assessment of older people: self-maintaining and instrumental activities of daily living. Gerontologist 1969; 9(3): 179-86.
[http://dx.doi.org/10.1093/geront/9.3_Part_1.179] [PMID: 5349366]

## CHAPTER 5

# Osteoporosis

**Tamara Pobocik**[1,2,*]

[1] *The State University of New York, Plattsburgh 101 Broad St. Plattsburgh, NY 12901, USA*

[2] *Saginaw Valley State University, University Center, MI 48604, USA*

**Abstract:** Osteoporosis is a silent destructor of bone. King, Clarke and Sandhu (2014) reported that as many as 10 million Americans have osteoporosis and this number will increase by 50% by 2025. This disease is not gender selective; however, women are the prevalent gender affected. Many do not consider this a problem; because one cannot observe the bone destruction until this disease progresses into advanced stages. Bringing forward information to both genders is an important preventer of this silent, but painful condition. Imagine presenting with a bone or spinal fracture that is not associated with any trauma or injury. This is a typical presentation for a person who has osteoporosis. Pain then becomes the driver of stopping the progression of this disease. As many times after a fracture, a person must deal with the acute pain of the fracture and then has the potential to become chronic pain for many individuals. Knowledge and prevention are the key factors to this devastating disease.

**Keywords:** Balance, Diagnostics, Fall risks, Falls, Gait, Osteoporosis, Rehabilitation, Walking.

## INTRODUCTION

This disease's characteristics are decreased bone mass, deterioration of the bone, and porous bone. Mackey and Whitaker [1] reported that osteoporosis is a progressive disease in which the bones become thin and become prone to fracture. A precursor to this disease is a condition known as osteopenia, and a screening test can identify this condition. Bone reaches its peak mass when an individual reaches the age of 30. After crossing 30, bones loose mass, they start to break-down at a rate faster than bone growth, and bone becomes spongy. When an individual does not maintain a proper diet, engage in weight bearing exercises, and avoid activities that slow or maintain bone structure then osteoporosis starts to occur. Individuals must maintain good bone health and it is never too late to

* **Corresponding author Tamara Pobocik:** Saginaw Valley State University, University Center, MI 48604, USA; Tel: 928 273 2122; Email: tpobocik@svsu.edu

influence and improve bone health later in life [2]. Nurses can make an impact on educating individuals on this destructive disease. In the Institute of Medicine Report [3], they recognized that nurses must practice to the fullest extent of their education. What this means is that nurses can improve health outcomes and reduce cost for patients in health care (IOM, 2010). As nurses are the primary education providers to their patients. This chapter will explore relevant information on osteoporosis for anyone who is interested to gain a stronger knowledge foundation on osteoporosis.

## Pathology

The pathology of bone formation is critical to understand how this bone destruction leads to osteoporosis. Osteoblasts, osteocytes, and osteoclasts are the three main components of bone formation in the human body. The marrow of long bones is responsible for the production of osteoblasts, osteocytes, and osteoclasts. Osteoblasts are responsible for the formation of new bone, and these osteoblasts then mature into osteocytes, which are the main component of bones. The osteoclasts are then responsible for bone resorption, which is how new bone replaces old bone.

This is a simplification of the normal process of bone formation throughout one's life. There is a positive balance of bone during childhood until peak bone mass is reached in early adulthood, with a subsequent period of stability and then a negative balance in older age with osteoclastic activity greater than production of osteoblastic activity, which leads to bone loss [4]. This means that after the age of 30, bones do not rebuild at the previous rate and without careful planning on how to increase the formation of new osteoblasts the disease process of osteoporosis begins.

Hormones in women influence bone formation. The female sex hormone estrogen plays a major role in the formation of osteoblasts. Tella and Gallagher [5] stated that a decrease in estrogen causes changes in the remodeling bone process. Women have time during their lives when this hormone fluctuates which eventually drops to minimal levels after menopause. Therefore, women at menopause have a decrease in estrogen, and are therefore the most affected gender of this disease. This is why educating women early can lead to prevention of osteoporosis. Another consideration is that some women experience problems earlier in life that can lead to low estrogen levels, for example amenorrhea, polycystic ovarian syndrome, being an athlete, anorexia, and bulimia [6]. Knowing the risk factors early can help to decrease the number of osteoporosis cases.

Other disease processes and treatments can lead to osteoporosis in both men and women. These include, but are not limited to celiac disease, rheumatoid arthritis, hypogonadal states, certain endocrine problems, and some autoimmune diseases. Knowing how these diseases can eventually lead to osteoporosis is important for individuals who may have any of the above diagnoses. These individuals must become advocates for themselves, as some care providers may only focus on the disease process and not the possibility that they could and will develop osteoporosis. Becoming active participants in their healthcare is critical for these individuals.

Taking certain medication can put individuals at risk to develop osteoporosis. These medications include anti-seizure, steroids, oral hypoglycemia agents, proton pump inhibitors, and selective serotonin reuptake inhibitors. Many of these medications people take on a regular basis, and they can obtain these medications with a prescription or without a prescription and could be from different care providers. Which means primary care providers may not even know their patients are taking these medications. This information is critical to stop or decrease the incidence of osteoporosis. Individuals must educate themselves and ask questions to care providers when they do not address the possibility of osteoporosis. Nurses must start to take the frontline to educate and identify individuals who may be at risk of developing this costly disease. These identifiable diagnoses and medications are very simple compared to the risk factors that the next section will focus.

## Risk Factors of Osteoporosis

Knowing the risk factors of osteoporosis is the best preventer of this disease. Unfortunately, many young women do not have a primary care provider during their 20's and into their 30's. As many young women do not have medical problems and usually seek care for obstetrics. Recognizing this problem now with the older population, could start to change the face of the disease. This could lead health care providers to address women at a younger age rather than waiting until osteoporosis causes a bone fracture. Therefore, providing information at any point becomes crucial. Bone formation is steady throughout childhood and into one's early 30's. Therefore, during this time an individual must consume adequate amounts of calcium, vitamin D, and obtain certain exercise. Presented in this section are the risk factors for both men and women.

There are both non-modifiable and modifiable risk factors for women and men. The non-modifiable and modifiable risk factors are in Table **1**. Individuals are not able to change the non-modifiable risk factors and must gain knowledge about what can influence whether a person will develop osteoporosis is important. However, the modifiable risk factors are the ones that individuals can change to decrease their risk of developing osteoporosis. Knowing these factors can help to prevent and stop disease progression, as many of these factors individuals can change to decrease or prevent the disease progression.

Healthcare providers should discuss these measures with patients any time they seek medical care. Kling *et al.* [7] stated that primary care providers are responsible for identifying patients who are at risk for osteoporosis, and the FRAX tool is a computerized survey that can identify those who might be at risk for osteoporosis. The FRAX tool is a questionnaire that patients fill out and then the provider can evaluate them for the non-modifiable and modifiable risk factors. Therefore, individuals' must understand the importance of preventive care. Chang, Hong, and Yang [8] used a computerized instrument to detect individuals who may be at risk to develop osteoporosis, and found this instrument did have statistical significance to identify patients. As the Healthcare Reform Act continues to come into light with the public, individuals need to understand they can become active participants of their medical care. This means initiating questions and seeking out preventative education that registered nurses in the community setting provide. As many healthcare providers do not spend the time patient's need for education. Nurses have the knowledge and influence that can change the painful outcomes of this devastating disease.

Osteoporosis has two different classifications: primary and secondary. An individual diagnosed with primary osteoporosis means that there are no identifiable reasons that this disease developed. These can include both the modifiable and non-modifiable risk factors in Table **1**. What this means is that many of the changeable items in the table above could prevent the disease for many. Secondary osteoporosis means that another disease process and/or the treatment of that disease contributed to the development of osteoporosis. These are the non-changeable items in the table above, and the medication(s) to treat a disease lead to the development of secondary osteoporosis.

Understanding these risk factors is important for both men and women, as they must be fully engaged in their own health care. Many healthcare providers see patients for a yearly physical or an occasional visit other problem and do not pay enough attention on the prevention of certain diseases, like osteoporosis. Patients must share information with their providers about over the counter medications they may be taking, because sometimes they feel these medications are not important to share with a provider. Having nurses in care providers' office will be critical for decreasing and identifying those individuals who might be at risk. A nurse can take the time to obtain an extensive health and medication histories from patients during an office visit.

**Table 1. Risk factors for osteoporosis.**

| | Examples |
|---|---|
| | Poor nutrition |
| | Alcohol > 3 drinks a day |
| | Antacids |
| | Excess vitamin A |
| **Risk Factors (Modifiable or Changeable)** | Risk/Frequent falls |
| | Excess caffeine |
| | Increase salt |
| | Lack of physical activity |
| | Low body mass index |
| | Smoking and second hand smoke |
| | **Examples** |
| | Female gender |
| | Age |
| | Family History |
| **Risk Factors (Non Modifiable or Non-Changeable)** | Previous Bone Fracture |
| | Genetic or Medical Disorders |
| | Race/Ethnicity |
| | Long term use of steroids |
| | Menopause |

## Common Presentations

Many individuals seek care when they experience acute pain from osteoporosis and then find out they have some type of bone fracture. Mackey and Whitaker [1] reported that hip, spine, and wrist fractures are the most common in patients. The most common fracture diagnosed in the emergency room is a vertebral compression fracture of the spine [9]. Other types of fractures are wrist and hip fractures, and these types are usually due to falls. Fractures might result due to a fall or lifting, but many just happen with activities of daily living. Therefore, an individual can fracture a vertebra just from lifting, coughing, or sneezing. Nevertheless, the question arises did the fracture occur after the fall or was the fall a result of the facture. The next step once the fracture is stabilized and the pain is controlled a provider will start to do other specific tests related to osteoporosis.

The diagnostic exam for osteoporosis is a dual energy absorptiometry (DXA) scan. The DXA scan's results are scores that range from +2 to -2.5 and is reported in a T-score. These T-scores are based on healthy 30-year-old female bones. Women 65 years of age and older should have this test done at least every two years. When a patient's T-score is less than -2.5 they have a diagnosis of osteoporosis. There is also a disease process known as osteopenia, and those scores fall between a -1 to -2.5. When the scores are in the osteopenia stage, this is a critical time to stop the progression of the disease to osteoporosis.

In addition, individuals can have a screening test done to identify if they are at risk for osteoporosis. This screening test can be done at any time and is useful for those who do not meet criteria for a DXA. This is for individuals who do not have any non-modifiable risk factors. This test is the peripheral test and individuals can have this done in many community settings to help identify those who should have DXA scan done in the near future. Prior to age 65 any individual can have a screening exam; these are done at many community based screening programs.

## Cost of Osteoporosis

Cost is a consideration when reporting on the disease of osteoporosis. As noted previously in the chapter bone fractures are common with the diagnosis of osteoporosis. This alone can cost patients, insurance companies, Medicare, and Medicaid a great deal of money. Casey [10] reported that the cost of osteoporosis includes hospital care, social services, rehabilitation, long-term care, and medications of treatment. Patience [2] states that a fracture that occurs do to osteoporosis has associated mortality and morbidity risk and are costly in the medical, social, and personal realms. Educating on the prevention of this disease is the key to decreasing the cost to all stakeholders.

Nurses in community settings have the power to change the cost of this devastating disease. Planning screening events to encourage members of the community to attend will provide members with information not only their risk factors, but with disease information, and actual screening schedule recommendations. With these educational events, the cost of the disease can be contained. Other members of the healthcare team that can help to prevent this disease are physical therapists. They can instruct individuals on the best exercises to prevent this disease from starting and control the progression. With the Health Care Reform Act, individuals other than care providers have a greater influence on this devastating disease.

## Interventions

The best intervention is preventing this disease and for this individuals must perform specific types of exercises and eat certain foods. All individuals need to have 30 minutes of weight bearing exercise at least five days a week. Weight bearing exercise is activity that puts weight on the bones. According to Taylor [11] some of the best weight bearing exercise includes yoga, tai chi, brisk walking, golf, dancing, hiking, racquet sports, and strength training. Finding one or more of these exercises that is enjoyable is key to keep motivated. Without these types of exercise, the bones are at risk to thin and that is when osteoporosis develops. Another early intervention is eating foods that deliver adequate amounts of calcium and vitamin D.

Choosing adequate servings of foods high in calcium should be something that all individuals focus on throughout life. As described earlier bone mass starts to maintain and not build bone as readily at around age 30, so starting this early in life is crucial. The best source of calcium is finding foods high in calcium and the daily recommend amount is 1000 mg up to age 50 and 1200 mg after age 50 years old. However, Mackey and Whitaker [1] reported that too much calcium could lead to kidney stones, cardiovascular events, and stroke. So, education on these supplements is critical for patients. The amount of vitamin D is constant at 600 iu daily for all, and increases to 800 iu for those over age 70.

If an individual already has osteopenia or osteoporosis, they need to find exercises that do not create a risk of falling. They may need to build muscle mass and strength and then they may be able to progress to different activities. This strengthening can help with balance, because aging and deconditioning can lead to weak muscles that can lead to falls. This is where a physical therapist can help patients with appropriate exercises to build strength to prevent further falls. Another consideration is taking medications that are prescribed for the treatment of the disease, and this is discussed in depth in a following section.

## Diet Considerations

As noted in the intervention section calcium and vitamin D are crucial to preventing and controlling osteoporosis. Individuals must consciously plan to consume adequate amounts of this fat-soluble vitamin and mineral. It is important to start consuming these foods at a young age and continue through one's lifetime. This can be difficult for some who have lactose intolerance, and these individuals might need to focus on taking supplements. Leaning to read food labels and knowing the amounts of calcium in foods can help to ensure one is obtaining adequate amounts of both calcium and vitamin D.

Calcium a mineral that many different foods contain and some food manufactures have fortified foods with calcium. Remember that individuals under age 50 need 1000 mg of calcium daily, and the best source is through natural foods. Those individuals over the age of 50 need 1200 mg daily. Some foods high in calcium include; dairy, oatmeal, soy products, broccoli, sardines, salmon, orange juice with calcium, pasta, and cereal. To ensure that enough calcium is digested one must read food labels and count their daily intake. As this might mean individuals must choose foods just because they are high in calcium.

Vitamin D, which is a fat-soluble vitamin is not that easy for an individual to receive adequate amounts naturally in foods. The only foods that have vitamin D include milk fortified with vitamin D, fatty fish, and eggs. Because this is a fat-soluble vitamin, it can be stored in the fatty tissues in the body, so when the body needs help with the absorption of calcium these stores of vitamin D are available. Another source of vitamin D is from sunlight, so individuals who live in the northern areas have times of the year when they might not have exposure to the sun and therefore do not have the proper amounts of this vitamin. There are supplemental vitamins that individuals might need to take on a daily basis to ensure that proper amounts (600 iu for those under age 50 and 800 iu for those over age 50).

**Treatment**

When an individual receives a diagnosis of osteopenia or osteoporosis, a care provider will likely prescribe medications. Two supplements that patients should take are calcium and vitamin D, and these are both can be purchased over the counter. With osteopenia the goal for the patient will be to prevent this from advancing to osteoporosis. Most prescription medications for osteoporosis fall into the classification of antiresorptive medications, and this means they slow the loss of bone. For a diagnosis of osteopenia, medications from the antiresorptive class are the medications of choice. However, with a diagnosis of osteoporosis the care provider might prescribed a medication from the bone stimulatory or anabolic class, which increases bone formation. In review, medications fall into two categories, and they are antiresorptive agents and bone stimulatory agents.

Antiresorptive agents include many different medications, and providers choose the medication that is the best for each individual patient. These medications come in different forms, that include nasal sprays, oral, and injection. The medications have varying instructions on the timing of the mediation in relation to food intake. In some medications the instructions are that, a person needs to sit upright for 30 minutes after taking the medication, as they can produce an irritation to the esophagus and stomach and lead to ulcers. These side effects and instructions might prevent some patients to take the medication.

The other class of medications is the Anabolic or bone stimulatory. These medications are injectable, and stimulate bone formation. Currently, this class only has a single drug called teriparatide (Forteo) and is a daily subcutaneous injection. There are two new drugs on the horizon in this classification and in clinical trials they are showing great promise, and are likely to become the gold standard for treatment of osteoporosis [5]. These drugs neither have the side effects nor complex administration instructions. However, individuals must learn to give themselves injections.

Some care providers might recommend that patients take medications from both the antiresorptive agents and the bone stimulatory group. A meta-analysis study, the authors concluded that there is no support at this time that this is an effective treatment option [12]. Another study done by Karlsoon *et al.* [13] noted that patients who were taking an injectable form of antiresorptive agents were more compliant than those taking oral forms. During this consideration process the provider will review other medications the patient might be taking, as this process can help a patient understand the importance of the medication. When this occurs the patient has an ownership of the responsibilities, their own lifestyle preferences, and comfort with administration should all be taken into consideration.

**Psychological Information**

Osteoporosis can be a devastating diagnosis for individuals, as the treatments are costly, chronic pain can be an issue, and individuals must modify their lifestyles. Helping them with all of these issues can ensure individuals take the needed steps to ensure this disease process is halted. Understanding the importance of goal setting might be a way for people to take ownership of their own health. Nurses can be the healthcare professionals responsible for slowing this devastating disease. Working with patients in outpatient settings nurses can provide one on one goal setting sessions to help each patient to identify how they could change eating preferences, exercise habits, and medication administration.

Individuals must have good support systems not only in the healthcare setting, but also in their personal lives. Understanding that the treatment of this complex disease can be time consuming for patients, so bringing a support person to all visits can help patients, to ensure they retain the information provided. When an individual is receiving education he may not remember all the information and having a support person becomes important. Another consideration is for individuals who have been diagnosed with osteoporosis or osteopenia is to find a support group with others who have the same diagnosis. These are the ways that patients can increase their success in the complex treatment of this disease.

Osteoporosis is a chronic disease, which means that patients must understand that they must educate themselves on all aspects of the disease. Seeking clarification becomes important, as well as reading reliable information. Instructing patients to reliable sources can be done by nurses and other care providers. These could include books, pamphlets, medical, and government websites. Carne [14] stated that a good source for information on osteoporosis is The National Osteoporosis Society. Patients and care providers must work together to ensure that patients are following a plan that will prevent further bone destruction.

**Importance of Collaboration**

All healthcare providers must collaborate to bring awareness to osteoporosis. Nurses seem to be a good coordinator of care for patients, as they know all the different types and services of each of the different care providers. These providers include a physical therapist, occupational therapist, nutritionist, primary care provider, and social worker. Not every patient will need services from all of the above mentioned providers, but knowing how and when to connect with others providers can influence if patients seek advice on the prevention and treatment of osteoporosis. Each discipline has their own specialty and has different ideas and thoughts on this disease process. Primary care providers and nurses are two specialists that were discussed throughout this chapter, and the next sections will describe other members of the interdisciplinary team.

Nutrition as stated earlier is a critical concept for patients to understand, as they need to plan to find foods that prevent bone loss. A registered nutritionist provides information on the diet to ensure that patients know how to acquire foods with calcium and vitamin D [2]. Patients must be comfortable reading food labels and know exactly what they are looking for to ensure their vitamin and mineral are adequate in their diet daily. They may only need a few visits with a nutritionist, but should be able to easily contact the nutritionist if they have questions that arise later.

For individuals who have problems with activities of daily living they might need the recourses of an occupational therapist. When patients have a bone fracture they may not be able to care for themselves, and many times there are assistive devices for patients at home. For example, some patients might need equipment for dressing, or a device to help them in and out of a shower or tub, or utensils for meal preparation. Once the patients are taught how to obtain and use these devices they may not need to continue with regular visits to the occupational therapist, but will have information if further assistance required in the future.

With the cost of the treatment for osteoporosis a social worker can be a great asset to a patient. Social workers are a resource for patients; they can help patients identify services for community support, as well as help patients' navigate insurance guidelines and services to care. A nurse and social worker can work closely together to help ensure that a patient will have the resources they need with a diagnosis of osteoporosis. Social workers can also help patients when dealing with family and friends who do not understand the stresses of this chronic disease and the complex treatments. Social workers can be patient advocates when communicating with insurance companies.

## CONCLUSION

Understanding osteoporosis is the first step in preventing and slowing the progression of this disease. As only education can help individuals identify diet and lifestyle changes needed to decrease the possibility of 20 million people who will be diagnosed for osteoporosis by 2025. Changing diet, decreasing alcohol intake, smoking cessation, and increase weight bearing exercises are the simplest goals for individuals. Nurses working with patients to identify goals will be critical in the fight against osteoporosis. When patients have written goals this will increase the success of lifestyle changes. Finally, to increase the positive patient outcomes related to osteoporosis and osteopenia is to note that interdisciplinary collaboration is essential.

## CONFLICT OF INTEREST

The author confirms that author has no conflict of interest to declare for this publication.

## ACKNOWLEDGEMENTS

Declared none.

## REFERENCES

[1]     Mackey PA, Whitaker MD. Osteoporosis: A therapeutic update. J Nurse Pract 2015; 11(10): 1011-7.
        [http://dx.doi.org/10.1016/j.nurpra.2015.08.010]

[2]     Patience S. Promoting good bone health: how can we help? Nursing And Residential Care 2015; 17(2): 78-81.
        [http://dx.doi.org/10.12968/nrec.2015.17.2.78]

[3]     Ross AC, Taylor CL, Yaktine AL, Eds. Dietary reference intakes for calcium and Vitamin D. Institute of medicine (US) committee to review dietary reference intakes for Vitamin D and Calcium. Washington (DC): National Academies Press (US) 2011; 3. Overview of Vitamin D. Retrieved from: http://www.ncbi.nlm.nih.gov/books/NBK56061/

[4]     Curtis EM, Moon RJ, Dennison EM, Harvey NC, Cooper C. Recent advances in the pathogenesis and treatment of osteoporosis. Clin Med (Lond) 2015; 15 (Suppl. 6): s92-6.
        [http://dx.doi.org/10.7861/clinmedicine.15-6-s92] [PMID: 26634690]

[5]     Tella SH, Gallagher JC. Biological agents in management of osteoporosis. Eur J Clin Pharmacol 2014; 70(11): 1291-301.
        [http://dx.doi.org/10.1007/s00228-014-1735-5] [PMID: 25204309]

[6]     Fontenot HB, Harris AL. Pharmacologic management of osteoporosis. J Obstet Gynecol Neonatal Nurs 2014; 43(2): 236-45.
        [http://dx.doi.org/10.1111/1552-6909.12285] [PMID: 24502394]

[7]     Kling JM, Clarke BL, Sandhu NP. Osteoporosis prevention, screening, and treatment: a review. J Women Health (Larchmt) 2014; 23(7): 563-72.
        [http://dx.doi.org/10.1089/jwh.2013.4611] [PMID: 24766381]

[8]     Chang SF, Hong CM, Yang RS. The performance of an online osteoporosis detection system a sensitivity and specificity analysis. J Clin Nurs 2014; 23(13-14): 1803-9.
        [http://dx.doi.org/10.1111/jocn.12209] [PMID: 23876185]

[9]     Sendecki C. Osteoporosis: A concern for ed nurses? Canadian J Emergency Nursing 2014; 37(2): 31-2.

[10]    Casey G. Osteoporosis--fragile bones. Nursing New Zealand. Wellington, NZ 2015; 21: p. (1)20.

[11]    Kling JM, Clarke BL, Sandhu NP. Osteoporosis prevention, screening, and treatment: a review. J Women Health (Larchmt) 2014; 23(7): 563-72.
        [http://dx.doi.org/10.1089/jwh.2013.4611] [PMID: 24766381]

[12]    Li W, Chen W, Lin Y. The efficacy of parathyroid hormone analogues in combination with bisphosphonates for the treatment of osteoporosis: A meta-analysis of randomized controlled trials. Medicine (Baltimore) 2015; 94(38): e1156.
        [http://dx.doi.org/10.1097/MD.0000000000001156] [PMID: 26402797]

[13]    Karlsson L, Lundkvist J, Psachoulia E, Intorcia M, Ström O. Persistence with denosumab and persistence with oral bisphosphonates for the treatment of postmenopausal osteoporosis: a retrospective, observational study, and a meta-analysis. Osteoporos Int 2015; 26(10): 2401-11.
        [http://dx.doi.org/10.1007/s00198-015-3253-4] [PMID: 26282229]

[14]    Carne K. Osteoporosis and fractures: Diagnosis and management. Practice Nurse 2015; 45(5): 42-6.

CHAPTER 6

# Vision Changes and Ocular Disorders

**Jeremy W. Grabbe**[*]

*The State University of New York, Plattsburgh 101 Broad St. Plattsburgh, NY 12901, USA*

**Abstract:** Among the sensory changes that negatively impact older adults, changes in vision are the most salient. Problems with vision are associated with trouble reading and driving. The impact on activities of daily living is apparent and pervasive. Many older adults find that their lifestyles are most significantly impacted by visual changes and visual ailments.

**Keywords:** Accommodation, Diabetes, Retinopathy, Surgical correction, Vision, Vision changes, Visual aids.

## NORMAL CHANGES

During the aging process the eye undergoes a series of changes which are most pronounced by a loss of visual acuity. As one ages the crystalline lens starts to become more rigid and begins to acquire a yellow tint. Muscle fibers controlling pupil dilation start to break down and lead to a reduced amount of overall light entering the eye.

Many clinicians may note that some of their older adult patients refrain from driving at night. In normal, healthy younger adults it takes approximately 40 minutes to complete the process of dark adaptation. In older adults the process is long and usually incomplete. Large changes in dark adaptation occur for people over the age of 60. Older adults are considerably less sensitive to light under dark conditions. In addition to these changes in sensitivity to light under dark conditions, older adults become more susceptible to glare. This compounds the detriment to night driving.

Although a minor change with age that has minimal impact, changes in color perception may have some role in interaction with older adults. Older adults are

[*] **Corresponding author Jeremy W. Grabbe:** The State University of New York, Plattsburgh 101 Broad St. Plattsburgh, NY 12901, USA; Tel: 1( 518) 792-5425; E-mail: jgrab001@plattsburgh.edu

less sensitive to blues and greens. These minor changes to color perception may relate to discussions pertaining to décor and/or fashions. One anecdotal tale shows caution in misunderstanding minor sensory changes. A young clinician in speech-language pathology in a geriatric practice met a new patient. The clinician was wearing a blue-green blouse. The patient noted the blue color of the blouse. What followed was a debate between patient and clinician over the color of the aforementioned blouse. At the end of the exhaustive discussion the clinician was under the impression that the intransigence of the older adult in admitting to the color of the blouse was due to possible mild cognitive impairment rather than changes in color perception.

A common and well-documented normal vision change in age is presbyopia. This age-related loss in the ability to focus on close objects leads to farsightedness in older adults. This is easily accommodated with corrective lens and larger print materials. In the clinical perspective of vision changes and aging, an important point to consider is visual function and visual acuity. Hidalgo *et al.* [1] address this issue in great detail. Visual acuity is direct and easy to measure. In contrast, visual acuity may be corrected, but does not reflect visual function. Visual function encompasses the impact of visual acuity changes (*i.e.*, low vision) on activities dependent upon vision. Unlike visual acuity, visual function is more difficult to conceptualize let alone measure.

Hidalgo *et al.* [1] lays out the differences and problems:

Questioning older people about their visual problems may help in detecting visual impairment, however it is not as sensitive and specific as a direct assessment of visual acuity. By combining the scores of several questions, the sensitivity to detect visual acuity of less than 6/12 may be increased to 86%, but an assessment using a standard Snellen's chart is preferable. A systematic review of clinical trials, performed in older people in a community setting, included the assessment of visual function and concluded that evidence for effectiveness of visual screening was lacking, but a small beneficial effect cannot be excluded. In this respect the United States Preventive Services Task Force (USPSTF) recommends visual screening for impaired vision in people aged over 65 years using the Snellen chart (grade B recommendation). The Canadian Task Force on Preventive Health Care (CTF) points out that the high prevalence of visual defects in elderly people and the existence of effective treatment are sufficient reasons for including periodical visual acuity testing with a Snellen sight chart.

## OCULAR DISORDERS

### Cataracts

A common geriatric condition of the eye is a cataract. A cataract is a condition in which the lens becomes cloudy. This leads to blurriness of vision as well as an increase in problems with glare. Cataract treatment involves removal of the cataract. This procedure involves cutting away at the ectodermal opacity and replacement of the lens with a plastic lens.

Recently, Liu *et al.* [2] discovered a breakthrough in cataractogenises which is now leading to new ways to delay the progress of cataracts. In the lens the removal of damaged proteins is handled largely by the ubiquitin proteolytic system. The other mechanisms of removal are lysomal/autophagic mechanisms and calcium-activated proteases. The seven lysine on ubiquitin serve to remove damaged proteins although lysine 6 removes only a small amount of proteins. The research found that mutation of lysine 6 leads to high levels of calcium ions $(Ca^{2+})$. This also leads to hyperactivation of calpain and eventual to the onset of cataracts in the lens. Methods of exploitation of the ubiquitin proteolytic system and calpain-based degradative system are not attractive areas of exploration for the treatment of cataracts.

### Glaucoma

Another common ocular disorder among older adults is glaucoma. Glaucoma is an elevation of intraocular pressure of the vitreous humor. This prolonged pressure damages the neurons in the retina leading to significantly impaired vision. One of the first warning signs of glaucoma is a reduction in peripheral vision function. Often this goes unnoticed by the older adults until significant loss has occurred. This is because many older adults experience less peripheral vision processing due to contraction of the Useful Field of View (UFOV). The only exception is that the in older adults the Useful Field of View expands asymmetrically for word stimuli only [3]. This was theorized as a result of older adults' greater reading experience. A possible earlier warning sign of glaucoma could be if older adults report greater difficulty reading (particularly in reading speed).

The study of glaucoma and lymphatic defects in mice has resulted in the prospect of new treatments for glaucoma [4]. The authors found impaired ocular drainage in mice with a deletion of Angpt1 and Angpt2. This deletion resulted in a disruption of the signaling pathways for angiopoietin/TIE2. Angiopoietin/TIE2 plays an important role in the development of the lymphatic system. The mice did not develop drainage pathways in the corneal limbus. The authors note that these results offer "the intriguing possibility that promotion of lymphangiogenesis with therapies such as VEGFC or ANGPT/TIE2 agonists might represent novel and much-needed therapies for glaucoma" [4, p4323].

## Macular Degeneration

Older adults are at an elevated risk for macular degeneration. Age-related macular degeneration is characterized by specific loses within the visual field. These loses derive from drusen which are build ups in the retina containing extracellular material. Drusen often have a glittering appearance and are noted for resembling crystalline dots.

Age-related macular degeneration takes two forms: wet and dry. The dry form is characterized by the appearance of choroidal vessels near the fovea. In this dry form the specific loss of visual acuity/function in a specific area of the visual field is the first indicator of macular degeneration. The wet form of macular degeneration involves the detachment of the neuroretina from Burch's membrane due to hemorrhagic fluid.

De Jong [5] describes the stages of macular degeneration:

The stages of age-related macular degeneration are categorized as early, in which visual symptoms are inconspicuous, and late, in which severe loss of vision is usual. Early age-related macular degeneration is characterized by drusen or by hyperpigmentations or small hypopigmentations, without visible choroidal vessels. Drusen become visible on ophthalmoscopy when their diameter exceeds 25 μm. The larger the drusen, the greater the area they cover, and the larger the areas of hyperpigmentation and hypopigmentation of the retinal pigment epithelium (RPE) in the macula, the higher the risk of late age-related macular degeneration. Late age-related macular degeneration has "dry" and "wet" forms, but the question of whether these two forms are really the same disease is a controversial one. Both dry and wet age-related macular degeneration can be found in the same patient: dry age-related macular degeneration can occur in one eye and wet age-related macular degeneration in the other, or both dry and wet age-related macular de-generation can be seen in the same eye. In follow-up studies, dry age-related macular degeneration can become wet age-related macular degeneration, and wet age-related macular degeneration can become dry. Dry and wet age-related macular degeneration can resemble end stages of other retinal diseases, and for this reason, late age-related macular degeneration is a diagnosis of exclusion.

## Diabetes: Diabetic Retinopathy and Diabetic Macular Edema

In the field of aging vision research an important new relationship to explore is the connection between age-related macular degeneration and diabetic retinopathy. This has potential impact for opticians as well as those in the field of internal medicine. Diabetes mellitus has been documented to cause diabetic retinopathy. Although diabetic retinopathy and age-related macular degeneration are separate diseases, a relationship exists between the two. Recently Chen *et al.* [6] examined the role diabetes mellitus has in age-related macular degeneration. It has been a breakthrough in understanding the obscurity in the relationship between age-related macular degeneration and diabetic retinopathy.

Previous studies have found no correlations between diabetes and age-related macular degeneration [7, 8]. Other studies have shown links between diabetes and age-related macular degeneration [9 - 13]. What was important was the links between risk factors for age-related macular degeneration and the risk factors for diabetes. Smoking, diet, diseases, and age are all risk factors shared by diabetes and age-related macular degeneration. Diabetes may lead to higher levels of advanced glycation end products (AGEs). These AGEs show significant accumulations in the retina in both the photoreceptors and the retinal pigment epithelium. The high level of AGEs leads to an accumulation of non-degradable aggregate ligands. In people with diabetes these high levels of ligands have been found in macula in donor retinas with age-related macular degeneration.

Patients with diabetes will have hyperglycemia and dyslipidemia. Hyperglycemia is elevated levels of glucose in the blood stream. Dyslipidemia is an elevated amount of lipids (plasma cholesterol, triglycerides, and/or low-density lipoproteins). These conditions result in an inflammatory response in tissue culminating in oxidative stress. In comparing patients with age-related macular degeneration to healthy controls the AMD patients have reduced anti-oxidant capacity. The use of anti-oxidants and omega-3 fatty acids works to prevent retinal degeneration. It should be noted that these results occurred in animal models and to date the author knows of no known attempt to replicate these findings in human-subject trials. Oxidative stress in diabetic patients with age-related macular degeneration leads of inflammation and greater oxidative stress damage. Particularly, the inflammation response leads to the disruption in the regulation of chemokines and cytokines which lead to disruption and even necrosis of photoreceptors.

Looking further at the link between age-related macular degeneration and diabetic retinopathy, vascular changes become a factor in their commonality. In both diseases vascular endothelial growth factor (VEGF) leads to vascular complications such as ischemia, microaneurysms, and neovascular glaucoma. Anti-VEGF agents, such as bevacizumab, are a common treatment for both.

In a recent breakthrough, utilizing an Asian population from mainland China, has discovered better predictors for bevacizumab efficacy in age-related macular degeneration. Ma *et al.* [14] sampled the first non-caucasion majority sample to study anatomical and vision functionality. They found that early in treatment, observances of total macular volume and central retinal thickness. More startling was that total macular volume and central retinal thickness were more predictive of treatment outcome than best corrected visual acuity.

## Use of Vision Aids Prescription

With the increasing number of older adults who will have vision impairments, there will be the need for low vision aids. Approximately between 1-3% of the population of the United States and Europe are blind or visually impaired [15]. Many individuals with visual impairments are prescribed low vision aids (LVA) to redress problems with activities of daily living (see Table **1**). The Netherlands has an innovated medical initiative to provide LVAs to older adults. Such LVAs are closed-circuit television, telescopic devices, fluorescent, and magnification devices.

**Table 1. Advantages and disadvantages of different forms of visual aids.**

| Low Vision Aid | Advantages | Disadvantages |
|---|---|---|
| Stand Magnifiers | • Helpful with poor motor control<br>• Can be used with eyeglasses | • Trouble with bound books (unstable)<br>• Not very portable |
| Hand-Held Magnifiers | • Portable<br>• Adaptable to accommodate to different reading conditions | • Requires more motor control<br>• Often do not have light attachments |
| Magnifying Reading Glasses | • Spectacle mounted<br>• Hands free | • Require training/adaptation<br>• Possible eyestrain/headaches |
| Hand-Held Telescope | • Portable | • Require motor control<br>• Does not free up hands<br>• Limited field of view |
| Spectacle-Mounted Telescopes | • Hands free | • Distortion of depth perception and motion |

Despite the prevalence of LVAs, researchers have found that opticians were still more likely to prescribe optometric services such as spectacle-mounted aids over LVAs [15]. In particular, optometrists were significantly more likely to prescribe telescopic devices of the LVAs while multidisciplinary clinicians were more likely to prescribe fluorescent lamps.

## Types of LVAs

### Stand Magnifiers

Stand magnifiers work by means of a mounted fixed lens. The lens rest atop the stand and allows magnification of text. The benefit of stand magnifiers is that they do not require to be held. This allows for individuals with motor control problems to read efficiently. Stand magnifiers also work well with prescription eyeglasses. Also as they are stand mounted they are usually placed on a reading surface such as a desk and remain within easy reach. This has two distinct advantages for some older adults. If an older adult have range of motion issues an accessible and "hands free" magnifier is helpful to those individuals. The second advantage is that older adults with memory deficits benefit from the stand magnifier being in visual accessible. It then serves as a cue for recognition to utilize the LVA. Many older adults report numerous instances of forgetting to use visual aids. The greater accessibility of stand magnifiers serves to facilitate remembering to utilize the LVA.

### Hand-held Magnifiers

Hand-held magnifiers are easily portable magnification devices. They can be easily held in one hand. An advantage of hand-held magnifiers is their use when an older adults wishes to do some short reading such as a recipe or phone number. It allows for quick use as well as provides the ability to read at places other than a reading table or desk where a stand magnifier would be used.

### Magnifying Reading Glasses

Spectacle mounted aids are more commonly prescribed for older adults [14]. Magnifying reading glasses, as the name implies, are a device that is spectacle mounted. The distinct advantage of magnifying reading glasses is that they are worn by older adults. This frees up the hands which works well for individuals with motor planning problems. It also allows the older adult to more readily replicate the normal conditions of reading (*i.e.* sitting in a favorite chair and not holding hand-held magnifying glass or stooped over stand magnifier). In addition older adults are also able to preview a few more upcoming words than in the use of previously mentioned LVAs. Grabbe and Allen [3] found that for word stimuli older adults had a large preview window. This preview window allows older adults to compensate for age-related detriments in processing. A distinct drawback to magnifying reading glasses is that some training and experience are required to become proficient with them.

### *Hand-held Telescopes*

To observe objects faraway one LVA is the distance optical device often called a "monocular". This device is small and portable. It is useful only when remaining stationary. They also require excellent motor control. Individuals with tremors or poor grip strength have trouble utilizing these types of devices.

### *Spectacle-Mounted Telescopes*

In contrast to hand-held telescopes, spectacle-mounted telescopes offer hands-free use. This allows for the individual to move about while observing. Motor planning and grip strength are not factors for use. Furthermore, binocular and monocular enhancements are optional.

### *Treatments for Diabetic Retinopathy*

Surgical treatment for diabetic retinopathy is largely performed later in the pathology of the disease. This serves more to retard the progress of diabetic retinopathy rather than perform any corrective measure. The basis for deciding if a patient is a candidate for surgery depends upon visual acuity as a criterion [1]. The authors found that visual acuity alone is not a sufficient measure to account for the visual function of older adults with diabetic retinopathy. Furthermore, in the diagnosis of proliferative *vs.* nonproliferative diabetic retinopathy different criteria exist from different sources and ophthalmological organizations. The Royal College of Ophthalmologists of the U.K. [16]. defines the different criteria and diagnoses in Table **2**.

**Table 2. Retinopathy diagnostic guidelines.**

| ETDRS | NSC | SDRGS | AAO International | RCOphth |
|---|---|---|---|---|
| 10 none | R0 none | R0 none | No apparent retinopathy | None |
| 20 microaneurysms only | R1 background | R1 mild background | Mild NPDR | Low risk |
| 35 mild NPDR | | | Mod NPDR | |
| 43 moderate NPDR | R2 preproliferative | R2 moderate BDR | | High risk |

*(Table 2) contd.....*

| ETDRS | NSC | SDRGS | AAO International | RCOphth |
|---|---|---|---|---|
| 47 moderately severe NPDR | | | | |
| 53 A-D severe NPDR | | R3 severe BDR | Severe NPDR | |
| 53 E very severe NPDR | | | | |
| 61 mild PDR | R3 proliferative | R4 PDR | PDR | PDR |
| 65 moderate PDR | | | | |
| 71,75 High risk PDR | | | | |
| 81,85 Advanced PDR | | | | |

Legend: ETDRS = Early Treatment Diabetic Retinopathy Study; AAO = American Academy of Ophthalmology; NSC = National Screening Committee; SDRGS = Scottish Diabetic Retinopathy Grading Scheme; NPDR = non-proliferative diabetic retinopathy; BDR = background diabetic retinopathy; PDR = proliferative diabetic retinopathy; HRC = high risk characteristics.

## *Photocoagulation*

Photocoagulation, also known as focal laser treatment, is often a single session treatment. The end result of photocoagulation is to arrest the progression of macular edema by fusing vascular leaks in the retina. These vascular leaks allow for increased intraocular pressure due to fluid/blood increase in the vitreous humor. This procedure is used more often in cases of advanced diabetic retinopathy and does not generally return visual acuity back to baseline, but arrests deterioration of visual acuity.

## *Panretinal Photocoagulation.*

Another laser treatment for advanced diabetic retinopathy is panretinal photocoagulation (scatter laser treatment). Unlike focal laser treatment, scatter laser treatment involves a wide area laser treatment. This results in atrophy of new blood vessel which halts the increased intraocular pressure due to angiogenesis. This treatment requires several sessions, but has become a common and effective treatment of diabetic retinopathy. Previously, a wavelength of 577 nm was used, but new and better results are found at 532 nm with less risk of hemorrhages and choroidal neovascularization.

## *Vitrectomy*

This surgical procedure involves incising the sclera. A cannula is then inserted into the eye and fluid is removed. This procedure can be performed as an outpatient. Vitrectomy does not arrest the progression of diabetic retinopathy, but slows its progress.

Pharmacological Treatment for Diabetic Retinopathy and Age-Related Macular Degeneration.

## *Ranibizumab*

A promising drug therapy for diabetic retinopathy is ranibizumab. Ranibizumab is similar to bevacizumab. Its action works by blocking receptor sites for vascular endothelial growth factor. Ranibizumab has been found to reduce macular edema, but was not found to improve visual acuity [17].

## *Bevacizumab*

Bevacizumab is a common drug treatment for macular degeneration. It is a pan-VEGF inhibitor and has powerful effects. The structural difference between ranibizuamab and bevacizumab is that bevacizumab has two activation sites unlike ranibizuamab. Bevacizumab also has a longer half-life than ranibizuamab. Treatment with bevacizumab can have side effects such as dry mouth, cough, voice changes, loss of appetite, diarrhea, nausea, vomiting, constipation, mouth sores, headache, and cold-like symptoms. Currently (as of 2015) a research team led by Alexander Foss [18] is examining the effectiveness of different doses of bevacizumab.

## CONCLUSION

Visual complaints/problems are a common problem among older adults. These visual problems are among the biggest factors that impair older adults' abilities to be productive, independent, and enjoy the quality of life to which they are accustomed. Among the problems, older adult face with a normal age-related loss of visual acuity are many ocular disorders due to aging and other pathologies, such as diabetes. Although many treatments exist to slow the loss of vision, few offer correction or complete arrest of the disease. Future research, particularly pharmacological, holds the promise of new and innovative treatments.

## CONFLICT OF INTEREST

The author confirms that author has no conflict of interest to declare for this publication.

## ACKNOWLEDGEMENTS

Declared none.

# REFERENCES

[1]     Hidalgo JL, Martínez IP, Bravo BN, Pretel FA, Ferrer AV, Verdejo MA. Visual function versus visual acuity in older people. Ophthalmic Epidemiol 2009; 16(4): 262-8.
        [http://dx.doi.org/10.1080/09286580902999397] [PMID: 19874149]

[2]     Liu K, Lyu L, Chin D, *et al.* Altered ubiquitin causes perturbed calcium homeostasis, hyperactivation of calpain, dysregulated differentiation, and cataract. Proceedings of the National Academy of Sciences. 1071-6.
        [http://dx.doi.org/10.1073/pnas.1404059112]

[3]     Grabbe JW, Allen PA. Age-related sparing of parafoveal lexical processing. Exp Aging Res 2013; 39(4): 419-44.
        [http://dx.doi.org/10.1080/0361073X.2013.808110] [PMID: 23875839]

[4]     Thomson BR, Heinen S, Jeansson M, *et al.* A lymphatic defect causes ocular hypertension and glaucoma in mice. J Clin Invest 2014; 124(10): 4320-4.
        [http://dx.doi.org/10.1172/JCI77162] [PMID: 25202984]

[5]     de Jong PT. Age-related macular degeneration. N Engl J Med 2006; 355(14): 1474-85.
        [http://dx.doi.org/10.1056/NEJMra062326] [PMID: 17021323]

[6]     Chen X, Rong SS, Xu Q, *et al.* Diabetes mellitus and risk of age-related macular degeneration: a systematic review and meta-analysis. PLoS One 2014; 9(9): e108196.
        [http://dx.doi.org/10.1371/journal.pone.0108196] [PMID: 25238063]

[7]     Fraser-Bell S, Choudhury F, Klein R, Azen S, Varma R. Ocular risk factors for age-related macular degeneration: the Los Angeles Latino Eye Study. Am J Ophthalmol 2010; 149(5): 735-40.
        [http://dx.doi.org/10.1016/j.ajo.2009.11.013] [PMID: 20138605]

[8]     Xu L, Xie XW, Wang YX, Jonas JB. Ocular and systemic factors associated with diabetes mellitus in the adult population in rural and urban China. The Beijing Eye Study. Eye (Lond) 2009; 23(3): 676-82.
        [http://dx.doi.org/10.1038/sj.eye.6703104] [PMID: 18259206]

[9]     Topouzis F, Anastasopoulos E, Augood C, *et al.* Association of diabetes with age-related macular degeneration in the EUREYE study. Br J Ophthalmol 2009; 93(8): 1037-41.
        [http://dx.doi.org/10.1136/bjo.2008.146316] [PMID: 19429584]

[10]    Borger PH, van Leeuwen R, Hulsman CA, *et al.* Is there a direct association between age-related eye diseases and mortality? The Rotterdam Study. Ophthalmology 2003; 110(7): 1292-6.
        [http://dx.doi.org/10.1016/S0161-6420(03)00450-0] [PMID: 12867381]

[11]    Karesvuo P, Gursoy UK, Pussinen PJ, *et al.* Alveolar bone loss associated with age-related macular degeneration in males. J Periodontol 2013; 84(1): 58-67.
        [http://dx.doi.org/10.1902/jop.2012.110643] [PMID: 22414258]

[12]    McGwin G Jr, Owsley C, Curcio CA, Crain RJ. The association between statin use and age related maculopathy. Br J Ophthalmol 2003; 87(9): 1121-5.
        [http://dx.doi.org/10.1136/bjo.87.9.1121] [PMID: 12928279]

[13]    Nitsch D, Douglas I, Smeeth L, Fletcher A. Age-related macular degeneration and complement activation-related diseases: a population-based case-control study. Ophthalmology 2008; 115(11): 1904-10.
        [http://dx.doi.org/10.1016/j.ophtha.2008.06.035] [PMID: 18801575]

[14]    Ma C, Bai L, Lei C, *et al.* Predictors of visual and anatomical outcomes for neovascular age-related macular degeneration treated with bevacizumab. Biomed Rep 2015; 3(4): 503-8.
        [http://dx.doi.org/10.3892/br.2015.448] [PMID: 26171156]

[15]    Burggraaff MC, Nispen RM, de Boar MR, van Rens GH. Optometric and multidisciplinary approaches in prescribing low vision aids-revised. Vis Impair Res 2006; 8: 17-24.
[http://dx.doi.org/10.1080/13882350600812502]

[16]    Diabetic retinopathy guidelines. London, UK: The Royal College of Ophthalmologists 2012.

[17]    Kobat SG, Turgut B, Celiker U, Demir T. Intravitreal ranibizumab injection in the treatment of refractory diabetic macular edema. Retina-Vitreus 2014; 22: 257-64.

[18]    Foss AJ, Childs M, Reeves BC, *et al.* Comparing different dosing regimens of bevacizumab in the treatment of neovascular macular degeneration: study protocol for a randomised controlled trial. Trials 2015; 16: 85.
[http://dx.doi.org/10.1186/s13063-015-0608-2] [PMID: 25873213]

**CHAPTER 7**

# Disordered Sleep among Older Adults

**Robert E. Davis**[*] and **Paul D. Loprinzi**

*The University of Mississippi, University, MS 38677, USA*

**Abstract:** The National Sleep Foundation (NSF) recommends that the average adult accrue between 7 and 9 hours of quality sleep per night for optimal health and performance outcomes; for older adults the recommendation becomes 7 to 8 hours per night [1]. The Centers for Disease Control and Prevention refer to insufficient sleep as a public health problem and, subsequently, recommend adequate sleep be considered as a vital sign of health. Lifestyle choices and personal habits often prohibit individuals from achieving this recommendation for healthy sleep duration, however, many adults fail to adhere to sleep guidelines because of an existing acute or chronic sleep disorder.

**Keywords:** Aging and sleep, Apnea, Sleep disorders, Sleep hygiene, Sleep research, Sleep stages.

## INTRODUCTION

Staggeringly, in America alone as many as 70 million adults may suffer from a chronic sleep disorder [2]. Sleep disorders are problems regarding an individual's ability to fall asleep, stay asleep, sleeping too much or at the wrong times, and exhibiting unusual behaviors during sleep [3]. Nearly 100 distinct sleep related disorders exist and each is characterized by one or more pronounced disturbances, such as, excessive daytime sleepiness, sleep efficiency, or the manifestation of abnormal events during sleep, such as, sleep disordered breathing or involuntary limb movements [2]. The more common sleep disorders include, but are not limited to, sleep apnea, insomnia, narcolepsy, and restless leg syndrome (RLS).

The diagnosis of sleep disorders comes from a variety of tools such as sleep logs, sleep studies, and sleep latency tests. The "gold-standard" method for the diagnosis of sleep related disorders is Polysomnography. Polysomnography is a sleep study in which brain waves, blood oxygen levels, heart rate, breathing, body positioning, and leg and eye movements are evaluated. In addition to the

---

[*] **Corresponding author Robert E. Davis:** The University of Mississippi, University, MS 38677, USA; Tel: 662-915-5521; E-mail: redavis1@go.olemiss.edu

**Jeremy W. Grabbe (Ed.)**

diagnosis of sleep disorders, polysomnography is also used to adjust the treatment regimen of those previously diagnosed with a sleeping disorder. This polysomnography testing can be done in an individual's home; however, it is typically conducted at a sleep center or hospital. There can be advantages to both the laboratory and home based testing. The hospital or lab setting provides a more controlled environment for testing to occur, however, the participant may not exhibit their normal sleep behavior when removed from their usual sleeping environment. Home based polysomnography testing can also present problems with the transition of equipment used for testing from the lab to the participant's home.

Researchers and clinical practitioners often utilize polysomnography to assess sleep disturbances and disorders because of the robustness of the data synthesized. At times however, researchers may use a variety of more subjective assessment devices which rely on the self-report of the individual being evaluated. Such subjective methods consist of survey instruments and sleep diaries which assess the effects of the sleep disorders (*i.e.* sleep disturbances). Although several validated instruments exist, one such questionnaire commonly used in research is the Pittsburgh Sleep Quality Index. Developed in 1988, the Pittsburgh Sleep Quality Index is a self-report assessment of sleep quality disturbances, where the participant is asked to recall sleep related events over a period of one month. Disturbances assessed include subjective sleep quality, sleep latency, sleep duration, habitual sleep efficiency, use of sleep medications, and daytime sleepiness [4].

*Sleep architecture* is a term clinicians and researchers use to reflect the usual pattern of an individual's sleep. Normal sleep consists of a cycle represented by 5 distinct stages which we continuously move through then repeat during sleep. Each sleep cycle lasts approximately 90 minutes and upon culmination reengages. The first 4 stages comprise what is known as non rapid eye movement sleep (NREM), with stage 5 reflecting rapid eye movement sleep or simply (REM) sleep. The majority of the sleep cycle is spent in what is referred to as NREM sleep and this distinction of the sleep cycle involves movement through 4 stages. The first stage is a state of light sleep where the individual is between a state of awake and asleep. In stage two the individual becomes disengaged from their surroundings and initiates sleep. Finally, stages three and four are the deepest and most restorative. REM sleep is the portion of sleep where the brain is aroused and dreams occur. Seventy-five percent of a sleep cycle is spent in NREM sleep while roughly 25% is spent in REM sleep.

Older adults are perceived as a vulnerable population in regards to sleep problems for several reasons. As much as 70% of elderly individuals may suffer from chronic sleep disturbances [5]. Research also suggests that women may be more vulnerable to disordered sleep than elderly males [6, 7]. Such findings are of public health concern as insufficient sleep is associated with increased cardiovascular risk and early mortality [8 - 10].

Given age group of interest there are several factors worthy of mention which could potentially influence the presence of sleep disturbances. Changes occur as we age which affect or disrupt natural sleep architecture, such as, changes in life related events. However, once reaching the status of "older adults" (typically viewed as 65+ years) chronological age does not seem to alter the presence or severity of sleep disturbances [11]. Regarding sleep architecture, older adults tend to spend more sleep time in the earlier stages of sleep (*i.e.* 1 & 2) and less time in the later, more restorative stages (3 – 5). Whether or not the individual has retired is one such specific event capable of altering sleep behavior. The individual's daily work/life balance changes, which can cause the altering of sleep behaviors. Some research shows a protective effect of retirement on sleep [7]. This is hypothesized to occur as a result of removal of the pressure of a structured sleep schedule.

Likewise, spousal presence/relationship may play an important role in sleep patterns among adults. Given the strong relationship between depression and sleep-related problems [12], one could theorize about the effect of spousal death on sleep quality. Research reflects modest evidence for an effect of widowhood on sleep behaviors [11].

Additionally, the age of this subpopulation places them at substantial risk for morbid conditions, for example, physical functioning loss, cardiovascular disease, diabetes, cancer, mental health disorders and cognitive decline [11, 13 - 15]. Numerous scientific studies have provided evidence which reflect a positive association between sleep disorders in the elderly and comorbid conditions such as those discussed earlier [11, 16 - 18]. Also contributing to sleep behavior changes and the development of sleep related disorders in older adults are additional biological factors, such as, reduced production of hormones and neurotransmitters responsible for regulating sleep, for instance, melatonin and serotonin [19, 20].

# ASSOCIATION BETWEEN SLEEP AND NEGATIVE HEALTH CONDITIONS

As previously mentioned, sleep disorders are associated with many other diseases and disorders among elderly individuals. Common in the literature is the relationship between sleep disturbances and certain health outcomes [21]. The following will provide a brief summary of known associations between sleep disturbances and these common morbidities.

## Cardiovascular Health

Prospective studies have linked the presence of sleep disturbances to the realization of future cardiovascular disease. A study by Quan *et al.* [22] followed 4,467 elderly individuals for a time period of 1 to 4 years ultimately providing an association between sleep disturbances and cardiovascular disease. Likewise, evidence synthesized through meta-analysis, which reviewed 15 studies creating a total sample of 474,684 male and female participants, exemplifies the relation between sleep duration and cardiovascular health. Both insufficient and excessive sleep duration were found to increase the likelihood of cardiac dysfunction with insufficient sleep increasing risk for coronary heart disease and stroke while excessive sleep associated with coronary heart disease, stroke, and cardiovascular disease [23]. Most studies included by Cappuccio defined adequate sleep as 6 – 9 hours, with one Japanese study citing insufficient sleep as ≤ 5 hours.

## Cognition and Mental Health

An emerging area of concern, exemplified by the vast amount of research interest, is the relationship between sleep disturbances and cognitive decline. Sleep duration, regardless of whether its evaluation is based on the feelings of the individual or on a more objective recommendation seems to correlate with cognitive dysfunction.

Cognitive decline occurs as we age and the development of cognition-related health conditions, such as the varying types of dementia, are an all too realistic threat to the health and well-being of older adults. A prospective study tracked 1,041 non-demented older adults (65+) for a three-year period, hazard ratios were then calculated based on those who did and did not develop dementia [24]. This study revealed those who subjectively self-reported less than adequate sleep time were 1.2 times as likely to develop dementia when compared to individuals receiving, what they felt to be, adequate sleep. Additional findings were that those reporting trouble staying awake during the day were 1.24 times as likely to develop dementia. A meta-analysis of 18 cross-sectional or prospective studies inclusive of 97,624 older adults from 14 countries, conducted by Lo., *et al.*, found that, after controlling for various confounding variables (*e.g.* medication use, health status, alcohol consumption), individuals who slept less than a reference group of normal sleepers had 1.40 times the odds of having poor cognitive function. Reference groups for most included studies ranged from 6 – 8.9 hours of sleep with most equivalent to 7-8 hours, which reflect appropriate sleep recommendations [16].

Individuals with certain forms of dementia, specifically Alzheimer's disease, show a reduction in REM and stages 3 and 4, also known as slow wave sleep, while increasing time spent in stage one and two sleep [25, 26]. Such architectural changes are hypothesized to be due to structural degeneration of the brain and forebrain. Unfortunately, these disturbances appear to worsen with disease progression as those with more profound dementia show greater sleep disturbances [27].

Several potential mechanisms have been hypothesized to explain the link between sleep disturbances and cognitive decline. Due to the means by which these investigations occur, much of the evidence for the hypothesized rational comes from animal-based studies. Hypoxia due to sleep disordered breathing is shown to increase apoptosis and hippocampal atrophy [28, 29], amyloid plaques in the brain and tau phosphorylation all of which are components of Alzheimer's pathology [30]. This hypoxia resulting from sleep disordered breathing has been suggested as a potential cause of cognitive decline to the extent of conditions such as Alzheimer's disease [31]. The amyloid hypothesis proposes that sleep deprivation increases the concentration of amyloid-beta in the brain [32]. This is thought to lead to cognitive decline as individuals with Alzheimer's disease show toxic levels of amyloid-beta in the brain [33]. Animal studies have shown that circadian rhythm disruption can impair hippocampal function, learning and memory [34]. The hippocampus is thought to be the brain center responsible for learning and memory, with research suggesting that poor sleep patterns lead to neuro-inflammation disrupting neurogenesis [35].

In addition to cognitive dysfunction, there is evidence to suggest that other mental health conditions have a bidirectional relationship with sleep disturbances. Such mental health concerns are depression and anxiety disorder [36, 37]. A cross-sectional study of more than 2,500 adults age sixty-five and older supports that individuals suffering depression or anxiety (as identified by the DSM-IV-TR diagnostic criteria) were more likely than their counterparts without such mental health disorders to experience sleep disturbances [12]. Additionally, a prospective study of more than 4,000 elderly persons identified depression as an important risk factor for sleep disturbances [21].

## Physical Functioning and Chronic Pain

Differences in sleep quality are observed for older adults based on their level of functionality. Physical functioning shows strong associations to sleep disturbances among this population. Through the use of polysomnography and actigraphy, a cross-sectional study of 2,862 community dwelling men found that total sleep time, sleep efficacy, hypoxia, and waking after sleep onset all to be associated with individual physical functioning. Physical functioning was assessed *via* measures of grip strength and walking speed [38]. Similarly, prospective research inclusive of male and female participants showed poorer actigraphy-assessed sleep quality with worsening functional capacity among activities of daily living [37]. It should be noted that the Martin *et al.* study utilized participants from an assisted living facility. Analogous findings were also exhibited among older veterans participating in an adult day healthcare program [18]. Often associated with functionality in this population is the presence of chronic pain. As should be expected, increasing severity of chronic pain escalates the likelihood of experiencing sleep related disturbances in older adults [39].

## EFFICACY OF DIFFERENT TREATMENT METHODS FOR SLEEP DISTURBANCES

Different methodologies exist for the treatment of sleep disturbances and disorders. Methods range from traditional pharmacological means to non-invasive methods such as sleep hygiene practices. The following narrative will summarize the efficacy for several popular treatment options.

## Sleep Hygiene

Sleep hygiene practices have the potential to improve the amount and quality of sleep through a variety of practical actions carried out by the individual. Sleep hygiene is essentially habits or practices the individual performs which are conducive to quality sleeping. These practices may include the avoidance behavior of things like napping during the day, watching television while in bed, reducing bedroom noise, eating, exercising or consuming stimulants such as coffee, nicotine and alcohol close to bedtime. Also recommended is ensuring natural light exposure, creating a relaxing routine to perform nightly, going to bed at an approximate time every night and sleeping regular hours. The National Sleep

Foundation, Centers for Disease Control and Prevention and many other health conscious entities recommend practicing sleep hygiene practices.

Research regarding sleep hygiene practices shows promise, however, there are concerns regarding the methodology of studies focusing on the efficacy of sleep hygiene specifically in older adults [40, 41]. According to a review of the public health significance of promoting sleep hygiene, much of the sleep hygiene recommendations are the result of clinically-based study or laboratory testing, therefore, further study is needed to provide conclusive evidence for their propensity to treat sleep problems among the general population [42]. Additionally, investigation into the effects of stimulating substances or behaviors (*i.e.* caffeine, alcohol, nicotine, and exercise) seem to be moderated by individual tolerance levels and habituation [42, 43]. A study of older adults examined the ability of sleep hygiene practices, specifically caffeine, nicotine, and alcohol use to differentiate 4 groups of participants. Groups were formed on the basis of (1) those with insomnia who complain of sleep problems, (2) those with insomnia who do not complain of sleep problems, (3) those without insomnia who complain, and (4) those without insomnia who do not complain. This study used a total sample of 426 older adults and found no statistical differences between those using the stimulating substances by group inclusion [44].

**Pharmacology**

Pharmacological methods are often turned to for the management of sleep disturbances among elderly age groups. Melatonin supplementation has been used to treat sleep disturbances due to its propensity to encourage adequate sleep and synchronization of the circadian rhythm [45]. Interestingly, melatonin may purvey additional benefit to the elderly beyond sleep related issues with no known side effects even when administered in high doses [46].

Prescription medication used to treat sleeping disturbances is commonly referred to as hypnotic medicine, which is a common treatment method for correcting sleep disturbances in older adults. With insomnia, for example, older adults are twice as likely to be prescribed hypnotic medication as their younger equivalents [47]. There are 3 basic classes of hypnotic medication; benzodiazepines, non-benzodiazepines, and sedative antidepressants. The use of hypnotic medication in this population may be problematic because of the potential for dangerous drug interactions, as many older adults take multiple prescription drugs daily. Moreover, benzodiazepines should be used with caution in this population because of side effects, such as, daytime sedation and increased likelihood of injury due to falls.

## Exercise & Sleep

Interestingly, current research shows an interest in exercise as a treatment for sleep-related disturbances [48 - 51]. A recent systematic review reported that regular aerobic or resistance exercise training improved the quality of sleep in adults age 40 and older [52]. These results were the synthesis of 6 randomized trials using exercise alone as an intervention strategy, most lasting between 10 and 16 weeks. In addition, acute exercise (4-8 hours before sleep) has been shown to increase slow wave sleep, the more restorative stages of the sleep cycle, and REM sleep [53, 54]. Likewise, regarding chronic or habitual exercise, research also provides evidence of a substantial benefit on sleep quality, in the form of increased slow wave sleep and total sleep time while reducing REM and waking during the night [53]. Similarly, among a sample of older adults age 65-92 years, slow wave sleep and memory task performance were increased over a two-week period consisting of a daily social and physical activity intervention [55]. Interestingly, this study produced sleep improvements through engagement in light intensity physical activity, as engagement in moderate to vigorous physical activity may be contraindicated among many individuals in the geriatric population.

## CONCLUSION

Older adults are an at risk population regarding sleep disturbances and disorders. The relationship among sleep disturbances and other significant health problems in this group of people is a cause for concern. Future research should attempt to better understand the possible causal links between sleep disorders and conditions such as cardiovascular problems and cognitive decline. Moreover, it is extremely advantageous that researchers continue exploration into behavioral methods of treating sleep disturbances, such as physical activity engagement.

## CONFLICT OF INTEREST

The authors confirm that they have no conflict of interest to declare for this publication.

## ACKNOWLEDGEMENTS

Declared none.

## REFERENCES

[1]    Hirshkowitz M, Whiton K, Albert SM, *et al*. National Sleep Foundation's sleep time duration recommendations: methodology and results summary. Sleep Health 2015; 1(1): 40-3.

[http://dx.doi.org/10.1016/j.sleh.2014.12.010]

[2]     Altevogt BM, Colten HR. Sleep disorders and sleep deprivation: An unmet public health problem. National Academies Press 2006.

[3]     Sateia MJ. International classification of sleep disorders-third edition: highlights and modifications. Chest 2014; 146(5): 1387-94.
[http://dx.doi.org/10.1378/chest.14-0970] [PMID: 25367475]

[4]     Buysse DJ, Reynolds CF III, Monk TH, Berman SR, Kupfer DJ. The Pittsburgh Sleep Quality Index: a new instrument for psychiatric practice and research. Psychiatry Res 1989; 28(2): 193-213.
[http://dx.doi.org/10.1016/0165-1781(89)90047-4] [PMID: 2748771]

[5]     Van Someren E. Circadian and sleep disturbances in the elderly. Exp Gerontol 2000; 35(9-10): 1229-37.
[http://dx.doi.org/10.1016/S0531-5565(00)00191-1] [PMID: 11113604]

[6]     Leger D, Guilleminault C, Dreyfus JP, Delahaye C, Paillard M. Prevalence of insomnia in a survey of 12,778 adults in France. J Sleep Res 2000; 9(1): 35-42.
[http://dx.doi.org/10.1046/j.1365-2869.2000.00178.x] [PMID: 10733687]

[7]     Marquiáe JC, Folkard S, Ansiau D, Tucker P. Effects of age, gender, and retirement on perceived sleep problems: results from the VISAT combined longitudinal and cross-sectional study. Sleep 2012; 35(8): 1115-21.
[http://dx.doi.org/10.5665/sleep.2000] [PMID: 22851807]

[8]     Loprinzi PD. Health-enhancing multibehavior and medical multimorbidity. Mayo Clin Proc 2015; 90(5): 624-32.
[http://dx.doi.org/10.1016/j.mayocp.2015.02.006] [PMID: 25863417]

[9]     Loprinzi PD. Health behavior combinations and their association with inflammation. Am J Health Promot 2015.
[http://dx.doi.org/10.4278/ajhp.141024-ARB-538] [PMID: 26158680]

[10]    Loprinzi PD. Sleep duration and sleep disorder with red blood cell distribution width. Am J Health Behav 2015; 39(4): 471-4.
[http://dx.doi.org/10.5993/AJHB.39.4.3] [PMID: 26018095]

[11]    Smagula SF, Stone KL, Fabio A, Cauley JA. Risk factors for sleep disturbances in older adults: Evidence from prospective studies. Sleep Med Rev 2015.
[http://dx.doi.org/10.1016/j.smrv.2015.01.003] [PMID: 26140867]

[12]    Leblanc MF, Desjardins S, Desgagné A. Sleep problems in anxious and depressive older adults. Psychol Res Behav Manag 2015; 8: 161-9.
[http://dx.doi.org/10.2147/prbm.s80642] [PMID: 26089709]

[13]    Abe T, Thiebaud RS, Loenneke JP, Loftin M, Fukunaga T. Prevalence of site-specific thigh sarcopenia in Japanese men and women. Age (Dordr) 2014; 36(1): 417-26.
[http://dx.doi.org/10.1007/s11357-013-9539-6] [PMID: 23686131]

[14]    American Heart Association. Older Americans & Cardiovascular Diseases. Statistical Fact Sheet: 2013 Update.

[15]    Kirkman MS, Briscoe VJ, Clark N, *et al.* Diabetes in older adults. Diabetes Care 2012; 35(12): 2650-64.
[http://dx.doi.org/10.2337/dc12-1801] [PMID: 23100048]

[16]    Lo JC, Groeger JA, Cheng GH, Dijk DJ, Chee MW. Self-reported sleep duration and cognitive performance in older adults: a systematic review and meta-analysis. Sleep Medicine 2015.
[http://dx.doi.org/10.1016/j.sleep.2015.02.078]

[17]    Mercadante S, Aielli F, Adile C, Ferrera P, Valle A, Cartoni C, *et al.* Porzio G. Sleep disturbances in patients with advanced cancer in different palliative care settings. J Pain Symptom Manage 2015.
[http://dx.doi.org/10.1016/j.jpainsymman.2015.06.018]

[18]    Song Y, Dzierzewski JM, Fung CH, *et al.* Association between sleep and physical function in older veterans in an adult day healthcare program. J Am Geriatr Soc 2015; 63(8): 1622-7.
[http://dx.doi.org/10.1111/jgs.13527] [PMID: 26200520]

[19]    Maggio M, Colizzi E, Fisichella A, *et al.* Stress hormones, sleep deprivation and cognition in older adults. Maturitas 2013; 76(1): 22-44.
[http://dx.doi.org/10.1016/j.maturitas.2013.06.006] [PMID: 23849175]

[20]    Melancon MO, Lorrain D, Dionne IJ. Exercise and sleep in aging: emphasis on serotonin. Pathol Biol (Paris) 2014; 62(5): 276-83.
[http://dx.doi.org/10.1016/j.patbio.2014.07.004] [PMID: 25104243]

[21]    Smagula SF, Koh WP, Wang R, Yuan JM. Chronic disease and lifestyle factors associated with change in sleep duration among older adults in the Singapore Chinese Health Study. J Sleep Res 2015.
[http://dx.doi.org/10.1111/jsr.12342] [PMID: 26412328]

[22]    Quan SF, Katz R, Olson J, *et al.* Factors associated with incidence and persistence of symptoms of disturbed sleep in an elderly cohort: the Cardiovascular Health Study. Am J Med Sci 2005; 329(4): 163-72.
[http://dx.doi.org/10.1097/00000441-200504000-00001] [PMID: 15832098]

[23]    Cappuccio FP, Cooper D, DElia L, Strazzullo P, Miller MA. Sleep duration predicts cardiovascular outcomes: a systematic review and meta-analysis of prospective studies. Eur Heart J 2011; 32(12): 1484-92.
[http://dx.doi.org/10.1093/eurheartj/ehr007] [PMID: 21300732]

[24]    Tsapanou A, Gu Y, Manly J, *et al.* Daytime sleepiness and sleep inadequacy as risk factors for dementia. Dement Geriatr Cogn Dis Extra 2015; 5(2): 286-95.
[http://dx.doi.org/10.1159/000431311] [PMID: 26273244]

[25]    Petit D, Gagnon JF, Fantini ML, Ferini-Strambi L, Montplaisir J. Sleep and quantitative EEG in neurodegenerative disorders. J Psychosom Res 2004; 56(5): 487-96.
[http://dx.doi.org/10.1016/j.jpsychores.2004.02.001] [PMID: 15172204]

[26]    Prinz PN, Peskind ER, Vitaliano PP, *et al.* Changes in the sleep and waking EEGs of nondemented and demented elderly subjects. J Am Geriatr Soc 1982; 30(2): 86-93.
[http://dx.doi.org/10.1111/j.1532-5415.1982.tb01279.x] [PMID: 7199061]

[27]    Bliwise DL, Hughes M, McMahon PM, Kutner N. Observed sleep/wakefulness and severity of dementia in an Alzheimers disease special care unit. J Gerontol A Biol Sci Med Sci 1995; 50(6): M303-6.
[http://dx.doi.org/10.1093/gerona/50A.6.M303] [PMID: 7583801]

[28]    Gozal D, Row BW, Kheirandish L, *et al.* Increased susceptibility to intermittent hypoxia in aging rats: changes in proteasomal activity, neuronal apoptosis and spatial function. J Neurochem 2003; 86(6): 1545-52.
[http://dx.doi.org/10.1046/j.1471-4159.2003.01973.x] [PMID: 12950463]

[29]    Nair D, Dayyat EA, Zhang SX, Wang Y, Gozal D. Intermittent hypoxia-induced cognitive deficits are mediated by NADPH oxidase activity in a murine model of sleep apnea. PLoS One 2011; 6(5): e19847.
[http://dx.doi.org/10.1371/journal.pone.0019847] [PMID: 21625437]

[30] Gao L, Tian S, Gao H, Xu Y. Hypoxia increases Aβ-induced tau phosphorylation by calpain and promotes behavioral consequences in AD transgenic mice. J Mol Neurosci 2013; 51(1): 138-47.
[http://dx.doi.org/10.1007/s12031-013-9966-y] [PMID: 23345083]

[31] Pan W, Kastin AJ. Can sleep apnea cause Alzheimers disease? Neurosci Biobehav Rev 2014; 47: 656-69.
[http://dx.doi.org/10.1016/j.neubiorev.2014.10.019] [PMID: 25451764]

[32] Landry GJ, Liu-Ambrose T. Buying time: a rationale for examining the use of circadian rhythm and sleep interventions to delay progression of mild cognitive impairment to Alzheimers disease. Front Aging Neurosci 2014; 6: 325.
[http://dx.doi.org/10.3389/fnagi.2014.00325] [PMID: 25538616]

[33] Tanzi RE, Bertram L. Twenty years of the Alzheimers disease amyloid hypothesis: a genetic perspective. Cell 2005; 120(4): 545-55.
[http://dx.doi.org/10.1016/j.cell.2005.02.008] [PMID: 15734686]

[34] Kondratova AA, Kondratov RV. The circadian clock and pathology of the ageing brain. Nat Rev Neurosci 2012; 13(5): 325-35.
[PMID: 22395806]

[35] Zhu B, Dong Y, Xu Z, *et al.* Sleep disturbance induces neuroinflammation and impairment of learning and memory. Neurobiol Dis 2012; 48(3): 348-55.
[http://dx.doi.org/10.1016/j.nbd.2012.06.022] [PMID: 22776332]

[36] American Psychiatric Association. Diagnostic and statistical manual-text revision (DSM-IV-TRim). American Psychiatric Association 2000.

[37] Martin JL, Fiorentino L, Jouldjian S, Josephson KR, Alessi CA. Sleep quality in residents of assisted living facilities: effect on quality of life, functional status, and depression. J Am Geriatr Soc 2010; 58(5): 829-36.
[http://dx.doi.org/10.1111/j.1532-5415.2010.02815.x] [PMID: 20722819]

[38] Dam TT, Ewing S, Ancoli-Israel S, Ensrud K, Redline S, Stone K. Association between sleep and physical function in older men: the osteoporotic fractures in men sleep study. J Am Geriatr Soc 2008; 56(9): 1665-73.
[http://dx.doi.org/10.1111/j.1532-5415.2008.01846.x] [PMID: 18759758]

[39] Chen Q, Hayman LL, Shmerling RH, Bean JF, Leveille SG. Characteristics of chronic pain associated with sleep difficulty in older adults: the Maintenance of Balance, Independent Living, Intellect, and Zest in the Elderly (MOBILIZE) Boston study. J Am Geriatr Soc 2011; 59(8): 1385-92.
[http://dx.doi.org/10.1111/j.1532-5415.2011.03544.x] [PMID: 21806564]

[40] Ellis J, Hampson S, Cropley M. Sleep hygiene or compensatory sleep practices: an examination of behaviours affecting sleep in older adults. Psychol Health Med 2002; 72: 156-61.
[http://dx.doi.org/10.1080/13548500120116094]

[41] Rodriguez JC, Dzierzewski JM, Alessi CA. Sleep problems in the elderly. Med Clin North Am 2015; 99(2): 431-9.
[http://dx.doi.org/10.1016/j.mcna.2014.11.013] [PMID: 25700593]

[42] Irish LA, Kline CE, Gunn HE, Buysse DJ, Hall MH. The role of sleep hygiene in promoting public health: A review of empirical evidence. Sleep Med Rev 2014.
[PMID: 25454674]

[43] Stepanski EJ, Wyatt JK. Use of sleep hygiene in the treatment of insomnia. Sleep Med Rev 2003; 7(3): 215-25.
[http://dx.doi.org/10.1053/smrv.2001.0246] [PMID: 12927121]

[44]   McCrae CS, Rowe MA, Dautovich ND, *et al.* Sleep hygiene practices in two community dwelling samples of older adults. Sleep 2006; 29(12): 1551-60.
[PMID: 17252886]

[45]   Pandi-Perumal SR, Zisapel N, Srinivasan V, Cardinali DP. Melatonin and sleep in aging population. Exp Gerontol 2005; 40(12): 911-25.
[http://dx.doi.org/10.1016/j.exger.2005.08.009] [PMID: 16183237]

[46]   Karasek M. Melatonin, human aging, and age-related diseases. Exp Gerontol 2004; 39(11-12): 1723-9.
[http://dx.doi.org/10.1016/j.exger.2004.04.012] [PMID: 15582288]

[47]   Stewart R, Besset A, Bebbington P, *et al.* Insomnia comorbidity and impact and hypnotic use by age group in a national survey population aged 16 to 74 years. Sleep 2006; 29(11): 1391-7.
[PMID: 17162985]

[48]   Loprinzi PD. Objectively-measured physical activity and sleep apnea among congestive heart failure patients. Int J Cardiol 2016; 206: 82-3.
[http://dx.doi.org/10.1016/j.ijcard.2016.01.038] [PMID: 26780681]

[49]   Loprinzi PD, Cardinal BJ. Association between objectively-measured physical activity and sleep, NHANES 2005–2006. Ment Health Phys Act 2011; 42: 65-9.
[http://dx.doi.org/10.1016/j.mhpa.2011.08.001]

[50]   Loprinzi PD, Loenneke JP. Engagement in muscular strengthening activities is associated with better sleep. Prev Med Rep 2015; 2: 927-9.
[http://dx.doi.org/10.1016/j.pmedr.2015.10.013] [PMID: 26844170]

[51]   Loprinzi PD, Loprinzi KL, Cardinal BJ. The relationship between physical activity and sleep among pregnant women. Ment Health Phys Act 2012; 5(1): 22-7.
[http://dx.doi.org/10.1016/j.mhpa.2011.12.002]

[52]   Yang PY, Ho KH, Chen HC, Chien MY. Exercise training improves sleep quality in middle-aged and older adults with sleep problems: a systematic review. J Physiother 2012; 58(3): 157-63.
[http://dx.doi.org/10.1016/S1836-9553(12)70106-6] [PMID: 22884182]

[53]   Kubitz KA, Landers DM, Petruzzello SJ, Han M. The effects of acute and chronic exercise on sleep. A meta-analytic review. Sports Med 1996; 21(4): 277-91.
[http://dx.doi.org/10.2165/00007256-199621040-00004] [PMID: 8726346]

[54]   Youngstedt SD, OConnor PJ, Dishman RK. The effects of acute exercise on sleep: a quantitative synthesis. Sleep 1997; 20(3): 203-14.
[PMID: 9178916]

[55]   Naylor E, Penev PD, Orbeta L, *et al.* Daily social and physical activity increases slow-wave sleep and daytime neuropsychological performance in the elderly. Sleep 2000; 23(1): 87-95.
[PMID: 10678469]

## CHAPTER 8

# Speech Language Pathology and the Aging Population

**Kate Hood**[1] and **Jeremy W. Grabbe**[2,*]

[1] *Sunnyview Rehabilitation Hospital, 1270 Belmont Ave, Schenectady, NY 12308, USA*

[2] *The State University of New York, 101 Broad St. Plattsburgh, NY 12901, USA*

**Abstract:** In this chapter, we will discuss the scope of practice in Speech Language Pathology (SLPs) specifically with the aging population, implications of the areas of communication, cognition, and swallowing due to abnormal aspects of the aging process, optimal services, and various therapeutic approaches to address those areas of communication, cognition, swallowing.

**Keywords:** Aphasia, Cognition, Dementia, Dysphagia, Evaluation, Oropharyngeal structures, Rehabilitation, Therapy approaches, Swallowing.

## INTRODUCTION

Speech Language Pathologists (SLPs) have been recognized as a type of therapists who address communication disabilities. We integrate our services with others in addressing patients ranging from birth to end of adults nearing the ends of their lives and their families. In the realm of neurogenic communication and swallowing disorders directed therapy services, the SLPs play a primary role in the screening, assessment, diagnosis, treatment, and research. SLPs are recognized as the only profession who are certified and licensed to treat communication disorders (speech, language, cognition), and swallowing disorders [1].

The educational background and clinical training prepare the SLPs to serve in a number of roles related to communication and swallowing disorders. The SLPs evaluate and treat disorders discussed in this chapter in numerous settings including, but not limited to: Skilled Nursing Facilities (SNF), acute care

---

* **Corresponding author Jeremy W. Grabbe:** The State University of New York, Plattsburgh 101 Broad St. Plattsburgh, NY 12901, USA; Tel: 1( 518) 792-5425; Email: jgrab001@plattsburgh.edu

**Jeremy W. Grabbe (Ed.)**

facilities, rehabilitation facilities, outpatient rehabilitation facilities, Home Health (HH) care services, hospice care services, children's hospitals, and even the school setting. Where the focus of the chapter will be on the adult population, some SLPs work with pediatrics who do experience a neurogenic communication disorder that may impact their speech, language, cognition, and or swallowing [2].

Evidence Based Practice (EBP) is the integration of research evidence with clinical experience/expertise and expert opinion to provide effective and high quality service. SLPs must use these rigorous criteria to judge the quality of research evidence in at least three domains: validity, importance, and precisions for their therapeutic practice. Judgments necessitate careful reading and evaluation of published studies, particularly their methods and results section. Studies with stronger methods provide higher quality evidence for practice than these with weaker methods. The highest quality evidence comes from a well-designed meta-analysis (quantitative synthesis) of more than one randomized control trial (RCT), whereas the lowest quality evidence involves expert opinions. However expertise option may provide important guidance for clinical decision. The importance and precision of study results are key components for judging the quality of research evidence for the SLPs. Most SLPs are familiar with statistical significance. However in EBP, that also matters in the clinical or practical significance of results as indicated by the importance of study outcomes, the magnitude of study effects, effect size, and the precision with which those effects have been estimated (confidence intervals). SLPs must be able to use the application of the research outcomes to practice with their particular populations or individuals. SLPs must assess the similarity of the study setting and participants to their own circumstances and determine the extent to which the study includes all relevant. Patient needs and clinical preferences must be given due weight in this process. SLPs need to continue to monitor the relevant significant literature for new evidence that may inform subsequent decisions [3].

The reason why SLPs have incorporated EBP into their therapeutic services is to ensure patients receive the best possible service informed by the highest quality of evidence available. This also assists with greater accountability and credibility to our role as provides. Incorporating EBP into our therapy also identifies gaps in the correct evidence, which may also permit the scaling up of research effort to generate high-quality evidence on key practice issues. The results from EBP should explain as to why certain practices work, and to provide a foundation for further innovation and change [4].

When the SLP is critically appraising the EBP, they are rating the overall quality of evidence based on the outcomes with the lowest level of evidence, balancing harms and benefits, balancing benefits and costs, rating the strength of recommendations, and suggesting implementation, evaluation, and updating strategies. When implementing decisions, SLPs must integrate research evidence, clinical expertise, patient values. Evidence does not make decisions. In fact, the same evidence may even lead to different decisions, depending on other relevant factors. However, it should not be assumed automatically that evidence is not applicable when the patients or setting are somewhat different than those in the studies providing the evidence. SLPs are careful to discuss possible options with the patient and/or family, including an explanation of how research evidence figured into the recommendations.

The purpose is to provide sufficient information to support an informed choice by the patient and/or family. Collaborative planning may also be required to refine the chosen option to suit patient or family preferences. The most successful implementation occurs when the evidence is robust and matches professional consensus and patient needs, the context is receptive to change with sympathetic cultures, strong leadership, and appropriate monitoring and feedback systems, and there is appropriate facilitation of change with input from skilled external and internal facilitators. Patients with communication and or swallowing disorders and their families stand to benefit if SLPs are successful in integrating relevant evidence into the clinical decision making [1].

Many changes occur in the body as we age, and should be viewed as natural changes. A sharp line should be drawn between normal declining abilities and deficits that are addressed by SLPs. Orientation will be intact for a normally aging adult, but it is abnormal for an adult not to be oriented to time, place, date, or even who he or she is. Healthy aging adults do not show changes in sustained attention tasks, but they do perform tasks more slowly than young adults performing the same task [5, 6]. Long term memory remains intact for the healthy aging adult; however healthy aging adults may have difficulty with short term memory and episodic memory [7]. An example of this would be that the healthy aging adult may remember childhood memories, but has a difficult time remembering recent events. The ability to process verbal language in daily life remains functional. Reading might be slow as compared to a young adult, but comprehension is still intact [8]. In comparing healthy aging adults to young adults with swallowing, it is normal to see the aging population to have a prolonged pharyngeal delay. Once the pharyngeal swallow is delayed with aging, the delay does not continue to increase as the normal aging continues [9].

According to WHO, people who have chronologically reached or passed the age of 65 have used the definition of "elderly" [10]. This phenomenon is also labeled as the "Silver Tsunami". The "Silver Tsunami" refers to the rise in median age of the U.S. workforce to high levels since the Social Security Act of 1935. It is projected by 2020, about 25% of the population with encompasses of older workers, who are over the age of 50. This large aging population will impact not only the US economy, but also public health and society [11]. Since the elderly segment of the population will rise from its current proportion of 13% to 20% by 2030, people with neurogenic communication and swallowing disorders, specifically those with dementia-associated communication problems will become one of the profession's fastest growing clinical population. By the year 2050 the number of affected individuals with dementia will rise to between 11.3 and 16 million. This will also become the most common single diagnosis for nursing home resides [12]. Aphasia is abrupt in onset, symptoms developing rapidly followed by slow improvement over weeks to years. Dementia usually is insidious in onset and develops slowly with gradually worsening from subtle impairments of memory, reasoning and problem solving. Dementia is a disease and not part of the normal aging process [13].

SLPs treat all people equally, however excellent clinicians determines through collaborative interactions with the patient, what the patient wants, needs, and determines what is possible [14]. There are many types of therapy services that are provided by SLPs: Rehabilitative/Restorative Care, Maintenance program, and Palliative/Hospice care. It is helpful to understand the meaning of these terms; however the focus of this chapter will be on the SLPs role in restorative therapy.

In the traditional role of providing therapy to treat neurogenic communication and swallowing disorders, SLP are asked to provide rehabilitation services. According to the World Health Organization (WHO), rehabilitation care calls for goals aimed at reducing impairment, increasing function abilities, and maximizing opportunities for social participation [15]. The goals for rehabilitation, specifically from the viewpoint of the SLPs, is to have the patient to regain as much speech, language, cognitive and or swallowing skills as possible, as much as their injury allows, and their needs drive them. The SLPs also need to teach the patient to compensate for the skills that they lack, and teach them to be in harmony with their lives [16]. An example of a restorative therapy goal would be "patient will be able to point accurately to single words from a field of 20 words on a communication board with 90% accuracy and minimal verbal cues".

In the maintenance program, therapy may be established after initial evaluation and a reasonable period of treatment determines that such a program would be suitable. The purpose of the maintenance program is to create a goal when further clinical improvement is unlikely. The SLP would design the maintenance program and after the program has been established and instructions have been given for carrying out the program, the services of the speech-language pathologists are no longer covered [17]. An example of this would be a therapeutic feeding program in conjunction with medical management may be indicated for a patient with an inefficient functioning of the esophagus during the esophageal phase of swallowing [18].

In the palliative care model of therapy, the SLP provides his or her own clinical expertise and develop strategies to assist with the comfort and ease to the patient's quality of life, to support family members in providing care for the patient, and to consult in responses in changes in patient's status [19]. SLPs roles for this particular type of service includes the following: consulting with patients, family, and members of the hospice team regarding choices in communication, cognition, and swallowing functions, consulting strategies and tools to support the patient's active participation in decision making including establishing their end-of-life goals, assistance in optimizing function related to swallowing to promote comfort and positive mealtime interactions with family members, and to become a collaborative consultant with members of the hospice team while providing input related to overall patient care [19]. A goal to reflect this particular type of therapy would be, "patient will use a communication board created for the patient, and as he points to "money" as a way to indicate concern about finances".

As SLPs who work with people with the diagnosis of aphasia, we remember many things when we interact with our patients. We as SLPs are preparing our patients for a lifetime with aphasia. As therapists, we remember to give fair assessments of prognosis, and stress the importance of the skills that have remained since the stroke. These skills can be used as scaffolding support from direct therapy approaches to treat their verbal nonverbal aphasia and/or indirect therapy approaches. Aphasia is a human disorder, meaning it not only affects language, but a person's life and relationship to others. SLPs never forget that we are treating a person with aphasia. SLPs provide active listening, but we also have boundaries in our profession, and need to refer to other professionals such as a neuropsychiatrist as needed. Last and most important, we are going to be counseling for communication disorders and not depression. Besides providing direct and indirect therapy approaches to address their specific aphasia, we also educate patients and their loved ones about their diagnosis, commonly used terms, and community based responses.

A typical scenario goes as followed for someone with a diagnosis of a left Cerebrovascular Accident (CVA). A patient is being assessed with a confrontational naming activity. For example a SLP has a patient who cannot say the word "brush." After 5 trials, the patient still cannot say the word "brush". The SLP will need to find strategies for the patient to say the word "brush". A bad therapeutic approach is to just simply name the object over and over. A good therapeutic approach would be to name a strategy to help the patient say the word. There are four widely used direct therapy techniques for aphasia, which are supported by EBP. They include Voluntary Control of Involuntary Utterances, Treatment of Aphasic Perseveration, Melodic Intonation Therapy, and Sentence Production Program for Aphasia.

The purpose of Voluntary Control of Involuntary Utterances (VCIU) is to improve verbal output in individuals whose speech is limited to automatic or stereotypic production of a few words or phrases. Gradually, involuntary (automatic) speech production is transformed into voluntary speech production-by using preserved oral reading as the "bridge" or "deblocker". The appropriate candidates for this specific program includes patients with severely limited speech (largely automatic or stereotypical) presenting with a unilateral left hemisphere stroke, comprehension superior to production, alert; oriented, good attention, and cooperative to therapy. The ideal patient must also match familiar words to picture objects and actions, and has at least inconsistent oral reading (for deblocking).

Theoretically, virtually all individuals with aphasia can produce some words under some conditions. Often these are words with strong emotional meaning produced in natural context. The goal is to identify the words/phrases that appear to be relatively accessible for the individual and help to bring those words/phrases under voluntary control. Ideally, the progressions of therapy involvement includes: involuntary utterances, oral reading (pair of written word with a symbol), confrontation naming, finally conversation level of communication. However, there may be a particular patient for whom the skill of conversation may precede confrontation naming. After a large number of words/phrases, about 200-300 words, have been achieved through deliberate effort, additional words/phrases should emerge as a result of deblocking.

Part of the VCIU program, SLPs must identify the words that the patients produced in some setting or another, and to determine which of these he/she reads correctly orally. These specific words should be printed on 3x5 cards. Additional words can be assess as a result of probing, and start with emotionally meaningful words. An initial set of words are selected and printed on cards. If the patient indicates fair consistency in reading the word, then it becomes a practice item. The printed word is associated with a picture or a symbol for confrontation naming practice. The printed word is gradually faded, while more words are added using the same process. Subsequently, attempts are made to elicit the words conversationally. To know when to continue with this particular therapy approach with the following guidelines, the SLP should be able to add at least one new word per session, patients should have some success with confrontation naming after 6-7 sessions, and should show progress each session [20].

Treatment of Aphasic Perseveration (TAP), improves functional language particularly naming by enabling the individual to deliberately control per-severative verbal behavior. In this respect, it is a "deblocking" program, in which the SLP is overcoming perseveration by increasing the accuracy of the language performance. Perseveration is pervasive in aphasia and may be a primary contributor to unsuccessful language attempts. There are three primary forms of perseveration in speech including: Stuck in set, Continuous, and Recurrent preservation [20]. Stuck in set preservation is an inappropriate maintenance of a category or framework of response after introduction of a new task. An example of this would be for the patient to sort a deck of cards rather by colors (black/red) rather than the new rule of even and odd numbers [21]. This is primarily associated with frontal damage. Continuous preservation is defined as an inappropriate prolongation or continuation of a behavior without cessation (*i.e.* mmmmmmmmmmm). This type of preservation is primarily associated with right hemisphere damage [20]. Recurrent preservation is an inappropriate occurrence of a previous response following the intervening presentation of a new stimulus. It is associated primarily with left hemisphere damage and most frequent seen in aphasia and is often elicited by confrontation naming task. An example of this would be the patient would be shown a photo of a key and say "key", but would say the word "key" to the next five common household items after. Apparent naming or word retrieval problems may be the consequence of perseveration-not primary naming or word retrieval problems. Therefore, treatment that addresses perseveration directly may not be effective. If the person lacks adequate cognition and self-control, then the primary goal would be to identify "set-breaking" maneuvers that communication could use effectively [20].

The goal of Melodic Intonation Therapy (MIT) is not to memorize a few melodies or intoned phrases, but to promote basic/functional expressive language *via* speech by using the linguistic resources of the right hemisphere, and to improve speech production or phonology [20]. Use of melody, stress, and rhythm may help mobilize the resources of the "nondominant" right hemisphere in the volitional production of speech used to encode meaningful language. This right hemisphere interpretation of the effect of MIT has been questioned based on PET scan studies of subjects undergoing MIT. The appropriate candidate for this participate therapy program would have a unilateral left hemisphere stroke primarily affecting the Broca's area of the brain. This specific aphasia would have the following clinical presentations: expressive language would be severely restricted, auditory comprehension would be at least moderately preserved, and demonstrates poor repetition. Automatic speech tasks would be evaluated as poorly to well-articulated. The psychological profile would need to be well motivated, aware of disability, and emotionally stable [20].

MIT's general principals of intervention includes, repetition, assurance of success, careful timing, avoid practice effect, and to avoid SLPs interruption. Therapy is designed to be intense with therapy completed twice a day for several weeks with family assistance. The key with MIT is to avoid familiar melodies which would tap into the patient's automatic language skills [20]. Criteria for continuation and advancement for MIT is for the patient to progress from one level to another. The patient must earn an overall 90% or better for five consecutive sessions using a variety of stimuli. Level 1: each of the steps (2-5) is worth one point; Level 2: steps 2-4 scored, 1 point if needed a backup to succeed, or if backup is not needed 2 points each; Level 3: 2-5 steps can be scored, 1 point if needed a backup to succeed, or if backup is not needed 2 points each [22].

MIT includes left-hand tapping and intonation. Tapping the left hand may engage a right-hemisphere sensorimotor network that controls both hand and mouth movements. It may also facilitate sound-motor mapping, which is a critical component of meaningful vocal communication. Furthermore, tapping, like a metronome, may pace the speaker and provide continuous cueing for syllable production. Intonation at the heart of MIT was originally intended to engage the right hemisphere, given its dominant role in processing spectral information, global features of music, and prosody. The right hemisphere may be better suited for processing slowly-modulated signals, while the left hemisphere may be more sensitive to rapidly-modulated signals. Therefore, it is possible that the slower rate of articulation and continuous voicing that increases connectedness between syllables and words in singing may reduce dependence on the left hemisphere [20].

## MIT Treatment Procedure: Step 1 (Elementary Level)

### Step 1: Humming

Therapist introduces the target phrase by showing a visual cue, humming the phrase 1x at a rate of 1 syllable/second, and then singing the phrase 2x while tapping the patient's left hand 1x per syllable

### Step 2: Unison Singing

SLP and patient sing the target phrase together while the SLP taps the Patient's left hand (1x/syllable)

### Step 3: Unison Singing with Fading

SLP and patient begin to sing and tap the target phrase together, but ½ way through, the SLP fades out while the patient continues to sing the rest of the phrase accompanied by hand-tapping, but no further verbal or oral/facial cues

### Step 4: Immediate Repetition

SLP sings and taps the target phrase while the patient listens. The patient immediately repeats the phrase assisted only by the tapping of the left hand

### Step 5: Response to a Probe Question

Immediately following the Patient's successful repetition of the target phrase (step 4), the SLP quickly sings the question (*i.e.* what did you say?) and the patient answers by intoning the target phrase. Hand-tapping is the only assistance [20].

## Treatment Procedure: Step 2 (Intermediate Level)

### Step 1: Phrase introduction

SLP shows a visual cue and intones the phrase 2x (1 syllable/sec) while tapping the Patient's left hand 1x per syllable

### Step 2: Unison with Fading

SLP and patient begin to sing and tap the target phrase together, but halfway through, the SLP fades out while the patient continues to sing the rest of the phrase accompanied by hand-tapping, but with no further verbal or oral/facial cueing

### Step 3: Delayed Repetition

SLP sings and taps the target phrase while the Patient listens. After a 6 second delay, the patient repeats the phrase assisted only by the tapping of the left hand. No verbal assistance may be given

### Step 4: Response to a Probe Question

Following the patient's successful repetition of the target phrase (step 3), the SLP waits 6 seconds, then quickly sings a question (*i.e.* "what did you say?") and the patient answers by singing the target phrase. No assistance is allowed [20].

## Treatment Procedure: Step 3 (Advance Level)

### Step 1: Delayed Repetition

SLP sings and taps the target phrase while the patient listens. After a 6 second delay, the Patient repeats the phrase assisted only by tapping the left hand. No verbal assistance may be given

### Step 2: Introducing Sprechgesang

SLP presents the target phrase in sprechgesang (* vocal technique between singing and speaking) 2x (accompanied by hand-tapping) while the patient listens. The word should not be sung, but instead, should be presented slowly with exaggerated emphasis on rhythm, and stressed (accented) syllables

### Step 3: Sprechgesang with Fading

SLP and Patient begin the target phrase together (with hand tapping), but halfway through, the SLP fade out while the patient completes the phrase alone

### Step 4: Delayed Spoken Repetition

SLP present the target phrase using normal speech prosody (no hand tapping) while the patient listens. After a 6 second delay, the patient repeats the phrase using *normal* speech

### Step 5: Respond to a Probe Question

After a 6 second delay, the SLP asks a question to elicit the target phrase using normal speech. The patient answers by speaking the target phrase without assistance of any kind [22].

Sentence Production Program for Aphasia (SPPA) is to improve the ability of nonfluent individuals with aphasia who demonstrate agrammatism. Agrammatism is the inability for patients with expressive aphasia to speak in a grammatically correct fashion. Appropriate candidates for SPPA includes patients with speech output production of words and short phrases in which words such as articles, prepositions, personal pronouns, and verb inflections are omitted. The patient must be able to demonstrate good single word auditory comprehension and fair-good comprehension for sentence and paragraphs. The patient may be frustrated by restricted ability to communicate, but is cooperative, has good attention span, and appreciates the goal of the program. SLPs focus would be to close the gap between what they need and want to make statements, requests, ask questions, and social commentary. Theoretical assumption of this treatment should be based on a carefully analysis of the patient's own strengths and weaknesses. With practice, patients who are agrammatic might improve their ability to produce a wide variety of syntactically correct utterances for purposes of communication [20].

There is a published version of SPPA which contains all the materials necessary for implementing the program. Target stimuli, stories and pictures are found in a spiral notebook. SLPs must come to each session prepared with about 15 exemplars, stories, and pictures for each sentence type to be trained in that session and score sheets to record and score each response. It contains eight sentence types each having 15 target sentences presented at two levels of difficulty, for a total of 120 stimulus items. Level A-requires patient to repeat the modeled targets sentence in response to a question. Level B- requires the patient to complete the story using the target sentence without the benefit of modeling. When presenting a level A question, the SLP should pause just before articulating the target phrase so the patient's attention is drawn to that part of the narrative.

**Level A Question**

Their father has fallen off the ladder, so Lisa yells at Nick, *"Call 9-1-1"*.

Prompting patient: What does Lisa yells at Nick?"

When presenting a <u>Level B questions</u>: the SLP should end their part of the narrative with a rising intonation so that patients will feel obligated to complete the story.

**Level B Question**

"Their father has fallen off the ladder, so what does Lisa tell Nick to do?"

Once the patient have responded correctly to a Level A question, the Level B question is presented immediately. When the accuracy criterion level (85%) has been achieved in response to the Level B questions, the 15 items for each sentence type are presented again, using only the Level B probes, before progressing to the next step. Scoring and goals involves an accuracy of 85% of the possible points for a sentence type at Level A & B <u>before</u> advancing to the next sentence type. SLPs want to document not only the reduction of agrammatism, but the improvement of the length and syntactic complexity with functional words in formal and informal reports [20].

Direct therapy approaches can also be provided to nonverbal patient due to a left CVA. The greatest difference from this patient to the latter is that this specific patient does not demonstrate any verbal communication, but depends on nonverbal means of communication to convey a message to their familiar communication partners. Three well-known treatments include Visual Action Therapy (VAT), Communication Drawing Program (CDP), and Anagram, Copy and Recall have been used as direct means of therapy to address patient's communication needs.

Visual Action Therapy (VAT) involves patients with very severe receptive and expressive language impairments who may learn to respond to gestures to communicate basic ideas with gestures. This program is simply an organized way to help people with *severe* aphasia send and receive gestures for purpose of functional communication. The goals are to improve expressive communication by using gestures, reduce either limb or facial apraxia, and possibly create a self-cueing system for the patient. For patients with limb apraxia with severe aphasia, the goal is generally to improve communication. The patient must be alert; oriented; demonstrates good attention; and cooperative in sessions. There is a reason to believe that damage is so extensive that the individual's stored language system is lost, not just inaccessible. Therefore traditional stimulation therapy would predictably be ineffective. For the patient with facial apraxia and severe aphasia, the goal is <u>specifically to improve speech</u>. The ideal candidate must be classified with moderate to severe facial apraxia; alert; oriented; demonstrate good attention; and cooperative. The theoretical assumption with VAT believes that even with a patient with global aphasia, some researchers believe that there is some degree of preserved cognitive and linguistic ability to use a symbol system [20].

The regime for this therapy approach is once or twice a day for 30 minutes. Materials for this therapy approach should use seven real, meaningful objects and not toys, seven shaded line drawings of these objects, seven pictures of a simple figure using the object, and possibly some additional contextual props to help elicit the gestures. VAT scoring involves 1 point for fully correct performance; ½ point for correct, but greatly delayed or self-controlled performance; 0 points for all other behaviors. The total points for the step is seven; patient must achieve 6.5 to move on to the next level. If the patient regresses from trial to trial, then the program may not be appropriate for that patient. Demonstrated steps are not scored. The main belief of this approach is to use small step or task analysis with the understanding that comprehension precedes production. There must be mastery at each stage. The hierarchy would be object, picture, symbol, discrimination/identification before functional use [20].

## VAT: Sequence Level 1- Real Object:

1. *Match Pictures and Objects (7 Objects and Matching Line Drawings)* (Place objects on pictures, Place pictures on objects, Point to object, give a picture cue, Point to pictures, given an object cue)
2. *Object Use Training* (SLP models with all objects; pick up object and demonstrates its use, Patient does the same)
3. *Action Pictures Demonstrated* (SLP pairs object with action pictures then points to the picture and finally picks up the object and demonstrate it use)
4. *Following Action Picture Commands* (SLP holds up the an action picture, patient finds corresponding object and demonstrates its use)
5. *Pantomimed Gestures Demonstrated* (SLP presents each object (in turn) on the table and demonstrates it use in pantomime (*i.e.*, without objects))
6. *Pantomimed Gesture Recognition* (SLP places all 7 objects on the table, pantomimes the use of one; encourages the patient to pint to the corresponding object. Proceed through all 7)
7. *Pantomimed Gestured Production* (SLP shows each of the 7 objects in turn each time inviting a representational gestural from the patient)
8. *Representation of Hidden Objects Demonstration* (SLP places 2 objects on the table, producing a representational gesture for each turn. Hide both objects under a box. Remove one object and produce a representational gesture for the other)
9. *Production of Gestures for Hidden Objects* (SLP places 2 objects on the table and requests representational gestures from the patient for each. SLP hides both; removes one; invites representational gestures for the hidden object. Proceed through all 7 objects)

VAT sequence for Level 2 would be substitute action pictures for real objects; sequence for Level 3 would be substitute object pictures for action pictures

Communication Drawing Programs (CDP) are for patients with aphasia who are unable to convey a desired message through speech or writing to communicate, but instead through drawings. Candidates must have the inability to communicate desired substantive information through either speech or writing. They must demonstrate the ability to use a medium-point felt tip pen to copy one dimensional shapes, relatively intact visual memory, good visual attention skills, alert, cooperative, and willing to pursue a drawing program to improve functional communication. Materials include 8 ½" X 11" paper, medium felt tip pen, clip art on a computer (for the SLP who is not good a drawing).

CDP's 10 therapy steps:

1. Basic semantic-conceptual knowledge (*e.g.* hammer, toothbrush),
2. Knowledge of object color properties (*e.g.* lemons are yellow),
3. Outlining pictures of objects with distinct shape properties (*e.g.* t-shirt, apple, pillow),
4. Copy geometric shapes (*e.g.* copy: star, oval, pyramid),
5. Completing drawings with missing external features
6. Completing drawings with missing internal
7. Drawing objects with characteristics shapes from memory, drawing objects to command from stored representation (*e.g.* named pictures with distinctive visual features),
8. Drawing objects within superordinate categories (specifically named objects and draw),
9. Generative drawing-animals and modes of transporting people (draw as many animals as you can think of),
10. Drawing cartooned scenes (1-2-3 panel cartoon stories "what's so funny about the photo?).

When scoring CDP for all steps, 100% accuracy must be achieved before advancing to the next step. The ultimate goal of the CDP is for patients to be able to use drawings as a functional means of conveying messages, ideas, thoughts and feelings. The readers are invited to guess the intended messages [20].

Anagram, Copy and Recall Therapy (ACRT), is an approach used to improve spelling so that writing can be used as a means of everyday communication in compensation for speech output deficits. Candidates for ACRT, must be diagnosed with an aphasia and agraphia caused by stroke, severely impaired ability to communicate through writing, can copy words correctly, good single-word reading comprehension (picture or word matching), written confrontation naming, relatively spared visual memory, good candidates have no difficulty in forming any of these letters of the prompt "The quick brown fox jumped over the lazy dog". Patients must perform well (>75% accuracy) on any reading subtest of picture-word matching and produces some correct letter for some of the 15 pictures from the Boston Naming Test. The general idea is to close the gap between the inability to express oneself verbally and the need to communicate needs and ideas, and close the gap between the poor ability to spell and the need or wish to improve spelling abilities. Treatment should focus on words that the family members/patient that are most functional, and start with the shortest words with the most regular spelling.

There are 5 steps for ACRT

*Step 1: Written Confrontation Spelling:* 'Write down the word for this picture",

*Step 2: Spelling with Target Anagrams and Word copy:* "Arrange these letters to spell fish"

*Step 3: Selecting and Spelling with Anagrams and Word Copy:* present the letters and two bogus letters and ask the patient to "Arrange these letters to spell fish",

*Step 4: Second Attempt at Written Confrontation Naming:* remove all samples of the word, point to the picture and say "write the word for this picture". Evidence of generalization in functional written communication is a great ways to document patient's use of writing for purposes of functional communication. Examples of functional writing would include but not limited to writing notes, lists, written messages, sending e-mails and postcards [20].

Indirect therapy consists of a combination of caregiver and or primary communication partner education and training to assist with communication changes for their loved ones. Family education would be completed *via* a multitude of educational approaches including discussion, demonstration, handouts, checklists, and role play to understand concepts. SLPs can provide controlled experiences in communication in an environment in which patients and their communication partners can try out new behaviors or new ways of communicating. This is led by an SLP in a structured task in which each member receives appropriate strategies to his or her abilities to reduce frustration and overall communication breakdown [16].

Dementia is a major health problem primarily found in people 65 years of age or older. It is an acquired neurological syndrome associated with progressive deterioration in cognition, visuospatial skills, language, memory, emotion, and even behavior [22]. Language is less affected than cognition, memory and intellect in early stages. Communicative activities that require greater mental effort affect first and most dramatically. Language professes that requires little mental effort (grammar, syntax, social conversation) usually are preserved until the late stages of Alzheimer's [16].

In the early stages dementia and its effect on communication, patients may omit meaningful words (typically nouns) while talking in sentences and have difficulty understanding humor, sarcasm, and indirect and nonliteral statements. Patients in the early stage of dementia are adequate conversationalists, but tend to drift off topic, and repeat material that is unnecessary. Middle-stage of dementia, people will demonstrate difficulty naming objects, may frequently repeat ideas and may fail to greet communication partners. Conversations with patients in the middle stage of dementia become passive conversational partners, allowing others to set the topic, tone, and content. Late stage dementia characteristics are generally unaware of surroundings and context, and use little meaningful use of language. At the last stage of dementia, they are nonfunctional conversationalists. They fail to observe social conventions (*e.g.* greetings) and are insensitive to the conversational rules such as turn taking and eye contact [24].

In treating dementia, the SLPs help manage the patients daily routines and help families cope with dementia [22]. To ensure appropriateness of treatment programs, decisions about goals, techniques, and stimuli must be made in collaboration with patients, their caregivers, and other health care professionals. Clinicians can work directly with individuals who have dementia to facilitate cognitive-communicative function ("direct" interventions); or indirectly through environmental modifications, development of therapeutic routines and activities, and caregiver training. Direct interventions are designed and implemented by SLPs; however, all direct interventions should be taught to caregivers for use after individuals with dementia have been discharged from skilled SLP treatment programs. Direct therapy programs include, Errorless Learning, Reminiscent Therapy Space Retrieval Training, Memory Prosthesis, and Montessori Approach.

Errorless Learning Therapy is better with patients in the early- and/or middle stage of dementia. This approach uses errorless strategies than with traditional effortful learning strategies. It uses the patients' intact procedural memory for rehabilitation of anomia and memory deficits. This is done to maximize patient's success and minimize the possibility of failure. The rationale is to avoid the production of errors by the patient entirely. It is believed that when patients are producing a response in error, it increases their odds of future failures. Minimizing the number of errors is the primary role of the SLP [25]. The reason is that the effect practicing the errors, which increases the odds of future failures. However, in severe dementia, any gains produced by errorless learning are limited and short lived [26].

Reminiscent Therapy is often a group activity that is used to facilitate communication for in the middle to late stages of dementia. It is designed to capitalize on patients remote activities, which is preserved until the very late stages of dementia. Patients with dementia usually have mostly intact long-term memory ability to increase orientation and to facilitate functional communication. Semi cued conversation regarding significant historical events (*e.g.*, the 1969 Moon Landing) or memories from the patient's past experiences. This is meant to increase orientation and to trigger recall of pleasant long-term or episodic memories. Individuals with dementia usually have mostly intact long-term memory ability to increase orientation and to facilitate functional communication.

This activity approach combines verbal stimulations with visual and auditory materials such as photography, maps, newspapers clippings, music to facilitate and enhance communication among group members. Typically, the SLP asks each group member to talk about what they remembered about the topic. Patients and the SLP encourages and reinforces patients' contributions. Utilizing this arrangement stimulates patient's interaction and facilitation of social skills. Activities with Reminiscent Therapy could include sorting photos by topic, subject, type or date, make a scrapbook, pasting photos onto the pages and writing notes about the memory beside the photo, labeling old family photos so you'll have that information later on, and watching or listening to comedy TV shows, movies and old radio shows like "Who's on first" (Abbott and Costello) and "I Love Lucy" [27].

Space retrieval training (SRT) is defined as an approach that gradually increases the interval between correct recall of target items. In early dementia, SRT has been used successfully to retain functional information such as face-name association with friends and family and techniques for safe swallow. SRT is particularly well fit for targeting the establishment of very important and functional knowledge (family names, bathroom, and bedroom) and emergency situations (calling for a nurse). This has been used successfully with patients with Traumatic Brain Injury, Parkinson's Disease, and Dementia related to HIV [28 -

31]. It is an effective tool that therapists can use to help patients reach their goals in rehab therapy and is billable and reimbursable. This approach takes advantage of the procedural memory system and is success-based.

Candidates for SRT are patients with mild to severe dementia who have declarative memory impairments resulting from dementia, and who can engage in structured training tasks. Training sessions should be administered weekly or more often and should teach verbal response and/or skills needed by the person with dementia. Caregivers should be trained in the response and behaviors expected of the person with dementia. SRT may improve the acquisition, retention and generalization of trained information or skill and may provide for retention of learned information or skill for intervals ranging from 1 day to several months. Space retrieval is unlikely to improve global cognitive functioning or general memory functioning. SRT is considered to be a modality or an approach that therapists may use to help patients reach their goals [24, 32].

Memory Prosthesis therapy approach helps people with dementia compensate for impaired prospective memory. Pocket size checklists remind the person with dementia of scheduled obligations with the person can check off when the obligation is complete. Some help with declarative memory-usually personal information, life history timeline, or information for orienting the person to his or her surroundings (*e.g.* location, time). This is best for people who have dementia but who can read and retrieve items of information from printed material [33]. Portable memory aids are useful, however only if the person remembers to use the aid. Consequently, their usefulness typically disappears by the time the person is in their late stages of dementia.

The Montessori Approach connects past interest and skills with present spared skills. For patients with dementia, they are designed to maintain and enhance physical, cognitive and social abilities. Activities are designed to capitalize on preserved procedural memory abilities of a person with dementia by guiding the person through activities designed to enhance sustained attention, facilitate adaptive behaviors and encourage socially appropriate [34]. SLPs may want to encourage activities such as constructing words and sentences from anagram tiles, sorting pictures or objects according to specific rules, constructing design with colored tiles and reading stories and answering story related questions.

The most important aspects of Montessori's principles include: breaking down complex tasks into individual parts, arranging these individual tasks hierarchically from simple to difficult, and from concrete to complex. The SLP should also provide extensive cues to guide the individual and facilitate success, provide feedback about the accuracy and appropriateness of performance to minimize frustration and failure, and utilize materials that yield cognitive and sensory stimulation. A therapeutic goal when using the Montessori Approach would be recalling family member's names to increase communication and socialization in visits by obtain family pictures and have patient assist you in cutting and gluing them to "flash cards" with their names for face/name recognition practice and matching [35].

In regards to indirect therapy approaches, caregiver training is essential to facilitating optimal outcomes for individuals with dementia. Most caregivers lack understanding of how communicative functioning will be affected in the different stages of dementia, and would profit from periodic counseling as the disease progresses. For this reason, and the fact that caregivers have continual, and often daily interactions with people with dementia, SLPs should consider caregiver training in any dementia management program. Both the environment and everyday routines are appropriate targets for management to improve functional communication abilities of individuals with dementia. Indirect interventions, particularly caregiver training in communication strategies, are appropriate for individuals in all stages of dementia severity including life videos and communication strategies.

Caregivers and SLPs automatically change the way they speak when talking to someone with dementia in the attempt to increase the patient's comprehension or attention to speech. This is called "code switching", or altering of the way one speaks depending on whom they are speaking. Yet, some communication partners are ineffective when addressing a patient with dementia as if they were speaking to a small child. Appropriate code switching should be subtle. Communication strategies for caregivers speaking when communicating to someone with dementia includes: speaking slower, using shorter sentences, augment what you are saying with appropriate gestures and facial expressions, writing out words not understood, avoid abstract topics and use more concrete topics, using frequently used words and avoid jargon, repeating important points, rephrasing important information, give the individual with dementia plenty of time to process what is being said, and avoid teasing and sarcasm which often leads to confusion [2].

Life Videos are custom-made personal videos, or life history videos. The purpose is to provide an audiovisual presentation of relevant personal facts such as relationships and past events to increase orientation and decrease behavioral disturbances of the individual. Researchers have found that after viewing these life history videos, participants with dementia showed significant improvements on measures of cognition [36, 37].

When it comes to environmental approaches, the main clinical concerns are to help the patient manage his or her daily routine, and help the family cope with the progressively deteriorating dementia for which there is no cure [23]. In the early and intermediate stages, communication, memory, and behavioral management are targeted. In fact, SLPs and other clinicians have used linguistic stimuli, such as large-print signs, to indicate locations of importance, such as restrooms, bedrooms, and dining rooms. The techniques of using tangible stimuli and single-word cues are both consistent with the principle of capitalizing on cognitive-linguistic strengths in managing individuals with dementia. Increasing lighting; decreasing ambient noise; creating a home-like, culturally appropriate environment; and developing familiar routines are all among the recommended strategies for improving cognitive-communication skills and other functional abilities in dementia, using night lights, post signs on doors identifying which room is which, having an identification bracelet [24].

Swallowing disorders, also known as dysphagia, involve impaired execution of the oral, pharyngeal, and esophageal phases of the normal swallow. A dysphagia may occur by a neurological incident such as a stroke or traumatic brain injury. Dysphagia is not a communication disorder, however except for the esophageal swallowing disorders, which is handled medically; the SLPs are the recognized experts in the assessment and management of swallowing disorders. A dysphagia can be treated by an SLP with a combination of direct and indirect therapy procedures. In direct treatment, food and liquids are placed in the patient's mouth to shape appropriate swallowing. In indirect treatment, food is not involved and an exercise regimen is used to improve muscle strength in practiced [38 - 41].

Direct therapy techniques can be viewed in dysphagia therapy as compensatory strategies. Compensatory strategies generally involve less muscle work for the patient and do not fatigue the patient as quickly as some swallowing exercises. Compensatory strategies include postural changes, increasing sensory input, modifying volume and speed of food presentation, changing food consistency and or viscosity, and introducing intraoral prosthetics.

Changing the patient's posture would help improve the specific swallowing disorder that is being targeted in therapy. Changing the patient's head or body can be effective in eliminating aspiration on liquids [42]. The chin-up posture is used to drain food from the oral cavity using gravity. It is best for patient with reduced tongue control. The chin down posture involves having the patient touching their chin to their chest. This pushes the anterior pharyngeal wall posteriorly. With the chin down, the tongue base and epiglottis are pushed closer to the posterior pharyngeal wall [43]. Head rotation to the damaged side twists the pharynx and close the damaged side of the pharynx so that food flows down the more normal side [44]. The chin down and head rotation positions may be best for some patients to achieve airway protection. Head tilting is best for patients who have a unilateral oral impairment and unilateral pharyngeal impairment in the same side. The head is tilted to the stronger side. When the postural strategies are successful, in time the SLP would reassess the patient in a normal upright position to determine oral intake without using the postural strategies are necessary. There are some patients who will need the postural strategies permanently. Because swallowing involves greater muscles contractions than speech, it has often been said by SLPs that the best exercise for swallowing is when it can be done safely and efficiently [45].

Sensory enhancement technique includes increasing downward pressure of the spoon against the tongue when presenting food in the mouth, presenting a sour bolus, presenting a cold bolus, presenting a cold bolus, presenting a bolus that requires mastication, presenting a larger volume bolus, and thermal-tactile stimulation [46, 47]. These techniques would help increase sensory input such as bolus taste, temperature, volume, and viscosity. Thermal-tactile stimulation technique is designed to heighten oral awareness and provide an altering sensory stimulus to the cortex and brainstem. When the patient initiate the oral stage of the swallow, the pharyngeal stage will trigger more rapidly [48]. Measure of the effectiveness of these sensory enhancement procedures in increasing oral sensory input include duration of time command to swallow until initiation of the oral stage swallow, oral transit time, and pharyngeal delay time [49]. Pharyngeal delay time can be measured from participating in a videoendoscopy procedure.

For some patients, modifying volume and speed of food presentation will help to create a faster pharyngeal swallow. For some patients who have a delayed pharyngeal trigger, a larger bolus size may help enable that trigger response. For some patients with a weaker pharyngeal response who may have to swallow two to three times per presentation, taking too much food too quickly can result in severe collection in the pharynx and result in aspiration. Those patients may benefit from smaller bolus size and slower rate of intake [39]. Eliminating certain food consistencies from the diet should be the last strategy that should be done only if other compensatory strategies (*e.g.* posture changes, swallowing maneuvers, who cannot follow directions) cannot be complete successfully. The appropriate level of thickness in liquids and the consistency of foods vary from patient to patient. For an example, a patient who has a delayed pharyngeal swallow response may consume thick liquids and thicker foods more easily than liquids that are thin. Another patient may preset with reduced tongue strength, wand would consume thin liquids the easiest than thick, heavy foods. SLPs would need to work with the facility dietitians to define specific foods prepared that fit the appropriate viscosity/consistency categories [39].

Restricting oral intake for certain food consistencies can be difficult for the patient. 0 to 80% compliance rates in sample of 8 patients with dysphagia. SLPs estimates of compliance were twice as high (71.9%) as observed compliance [50]. One research resulted in up to 21% noncompliance rates with SLP recommendations [51]. One of the top reasons for the compliance issues with altering food consistency or viscosity was that many patients dislike thicken liquids and poor patient [52, 53].

Intraoral prosthetics can be an important swallowing compensatory strategy for patient who have oral cancer and who also have a significant loss of oral tongue tissue (>25%) or tongue movement. A palatal lift prosthesis lifts the soft palate into a closed position in patient with velar paralysis. A palatal obturator can be used in oral cancer patient who have a significant resection of the soft palate. A palatal augmentation can be used for patients who have a significant tongue resection or bilateral tongue paralysis. A palatal reshaping prosthesis contours the hard palate to interact with the remaining tongue where the tongue cannot make contact postoperatively [44, 54, 55]. The prostheses are made by a maxillofacial prosthodontist with collaboration from the SLP. Creation of these prostheses should be made four to six weeks post-surgery to prevent patient from developing poor habits for swallowing.

Indirect techniques include stimulation of the oropharyngeal structures and the adoption of behavioral techniques, such as those involving postural changes or the swallow maneuver. These include oral motor control and range of motion exercises, and swallowing maneuvers. Oral motor control and range of motion exercises can be used to improve the movement of the lips, jaw, tongue, tongue base, larynx, and vocal folds. The most common occurrences with patients are with the following aspects of the tongue: lateralization of the tongue during chewing, elevation of the tongue to the hard palate, and anterior-posterior movement of the midline of the tongue in the initial stages of the oral swallow for example. Exercises to increase range of motion with the tongue target the patient's oral transit [56]. Having the patient push their tongue against a tongue blade focuses on both the tongue's range of motion and strength [57].

If the patient demonstrates poor vocal fold adduction, the SLP may recommend the patient perform vocal fold adduction exercises. The patient is asked to bear down against a chair with only one hand, and to produce clear voice simultaneously. Then the patient is asked to perform an "ah" with a glottal attack on each vowel. The second set of exercises involves lifting or pushing with simultaneous voicing with both hands, sitting in a chair, while prolonging phonation. Several tongue based exercises help improve base of tongue base range of motion. The patient could be asked to pull their tongue straight back for one second, second exercises is for the patient to pull their tongue back and gargle, third exercises is having the patient pretending to yawn while also pulling the tongue back. The falsetto exercises targets the larynx to elevate as much as the larynx goes for swallowing. The patient is asked to slide up the pitch scale as high as possible to a high squeaky voice [39].

There have been numerous swallowing maneuvers have been developed to play specific aspects to the pharyngeal stage of the swallow under voluntary control. The supraglottic swallow exercise was designed to close the airway at the level of the true vocal folds before and during the swallow. This was designed for patients who demonstrate reduced or late vocal fold closure when swallowing [58]. The super-supraglottic swallow was considered an exercise for the patient who demonstrated reduced closure of airway entrance. This strategy focused on closing the airway entrance before and during the swallow [58]. The effortful swallow exercise was intended to increase posterior motion of the tongue base during the pharyngeal swallow [59]. Lastly, the Mendelsohn maneuver was designed to increase the extent and duration of laryngeal elevation, and thereby increase the duration and width of the cricopharyngeal opening and improve overall coordination of the swallow [60]. The Masako maneuver was also developed as a pharyngeal exercises for patients who were diagnosed with incomplete contact between the posterior pharyngeal wall and the base of the tongue. Strengthening the posterior pharyngeal wall aids in the speech and efficiency of the swallow [61].

## CONCLUSION

Based on EBP, it has been demonstrated that communication, cognition, and swallowing rehabilitation therapy combining direct, indirect, and environmental strategies can be successful treatment strategies for the adult population. Accurate diagnosis of medication conditions often requires procedures that increase the SLP's sensitivity to different aspects of the disorder. The advantages of the various therapy approaches into clinical practice as well as research standards are numerous would increase their utility even beyond the current apparent applications. In cooperation with the patient's physician, other healthcare professionals, the patient, and caregivers, the SLP can design a program that would be developed specifically for the individuals communication and or swallowing needs.

## CONFLICT OF INTEREST

The authors confirm that they have no conflict of interest to declare for this publication.

## ACKNOWLEDGEMENTS

Declared none.

## REFERENCES

[1]     American Speech-Language-Hearing Association. Scope of practice in speech-language pathology [Scope of Practice] 2016. Available from: www.asha.org/policy/

[2]     Manasco MH. Introduction to Neurogenic Communication Disorders. 1st ed., Burlington, MA: Jones & Bartlett Learning 2014.

[3]     American Speech-Language-Hearing Association.. Evidence-based practice EBP 2016. Available from http://www.asha.org/Research/EBP.

[4]     American Speech-Language-Hearing Association.. Evidence-based practice in communication disorders [Position Statement] 2005. Available from www.asha.org/policy.

[5]     Berardi A, Parasuraman R, Haxby J. Overall vigilance and sustained attention decrements on healthy aging. Exp Aging Res 2001; 27: 19-39.

[6]     Plude D, Doussard-Rosevelt J. Aging, elective attention, and feature integration. Psychol Aging 1989; 4: 98-105.

[7]     Naveh-Benjamin M, Hussain Z, Guez J, Bar-On M. Adult age difference in episodic memory: Further support for an associative-deficit hypothesis. J Exp Psychol Learn Mem Cogn 2003; 29: 826-37.

[8]     Connolly L, Hasher L, Zacks R. Age and reading: The impact of distraction. Psychol Aging 1991; 6: 533-41.

[9]     Logemann JA, Pauloski BR, Rademaker AW, Colangelo LA, Kahrilas PJ, Smith CH. Temporal and biomechanical characteristics of oropharyngeal swallow in younger and older men. J Speech Lang Hear Res 2000; 435: 1264-74.

[10]    World Health Organization. Definition of an older or elderly person , 2016 [Retrieved March 1st 2016]; from http://www.who.int/healthinfo/survey/ageingdefnolder/en/

[11]    Chosewood L. Safer and healthier at any age: Strategies for an aging workforce 2012. Retrieved from http://blogs.cdc.gov/niosh-science-blog/2012/07/19/agingworkforce/.

[12]    Bourgeois M. Effects of memory aids on the dyadic conversations of individuals with dementia. J App Behavior Analysis 1993; 26(1): 77-87.

[13]    University of California San Francisco. Normal Aging vs Dementia 2016. Retrieved from http://memory.ucsf.edu/brain/aging/dementia.

[14]  Rosenbek J, Leslie P. 1182: Ethics & Evidence in Practice. Session presented at the annual convention of the American Speech-Language-Hearing Association 2014 November; http://graymatter-therapy.com/evidence-based-practice-misunderstood/

[15]  World health Organization. International classification of functioning, disability and health ICF , 2012 [Retrieved March 1st 2016]; from http://www.who.int/classifications/icf/icf_more/en/

[16]  Brookshire RH. Introduction to neurogenic communication disorders. 7th ed., St. Louis, MO: Mosby 2007.

[17]  American Speech-Language-Hearing Association. Model medical review guidelines for dysphagia services 2004. Retrieved from http://www.asha.org/uploadedFiles/practice/reimbursement/medicare/DynCorpDysphHCEC.pdf

[18]  American Speech-Language-Hearing Association. Speech-language pathology medical review guidelines 2011. Retrieved from http://www.asha.org/uploadedFiles/SLP-Medical-Review-Guide-lines.pdf#search=%22Model%22

[19]  Pollens R. Integrating speech-language pathology services in palliative end-of-life care. Top Lang Disord 2012; 32: 137-48.

[20]  Helm-Estabrooks N, Albert ML. Manual of aphasia therapy. 2nd ed., Austin, TX: Pro-ed 2004.

[21]  McNamar P, Albert M. Neuropharmacology of verbal perseveration. Semin Speech Lang 2004; 254: 309-31.

[22]  H lm-Estabrooks N, Nicholas M, Morgan A Melodic intonation therapy program. Austin, TX: PRO-ED 1989.

[23]  Bayles KA. Management of communication disorders associated with dementia. In: Chapey R, Ed. Language intervention strategies in adult aphasia. Baltimore: Williams and Wilkins 1994; p. 542.

[24]  Bayles KA, Kaszniak AW. Communication and cognition in normal aging and dementia. Austin, TX: PRO-ED 1987.

[25]  Fillingham J, Sage K, Lambon RM. The treatment of anomia using errorless learning. Neuropsychol Rehabil 2006; 162: 129-54.

[26]  Ruis C, Kessels R. Effects of errorless and errorful face-name associative learning in moderate to severe dementia. Aging Clin Exp Res 2005; 176: 514-7.

[27]  Akanuma K, Meguro K, Mehuro M, et al. Improved social interaction and increased anterior cingulate metabolism after group reminiscence with reality orientation approach for vascular dementia. Psychiatry Research 2011; 1923: 183-7.

[28]  Bourgeois M, Camp C, Rose M, et al. A comparison of training strategies to enhance use of external aids by persons with dementia. J Commun Disord 2003; 36: 361-79.

[29]  Camp CJ, Malone ML. Mise en œuvre d'interventions de récupération espacée auprès de personnes atteintes de la maladie d'Alzheimer. Cahiers de la Fondation Médéric Alzheimer 2008; p. 3.

[30]  Malone ML, Skrajner MJ, Camp CJ, Neundorfer M, Gorzelle GJ. Research in practice II: Spaced-retrieval, a memory intervention. Alzheimers Care Q 2007; 81: 65-74.

[31]  Neundorfer M, Camp C, Lee M, Skrajner M, Malone M, Carr J. Compensating for cognitive deficits in persons aged 50 and over with HIV/AIDS: A Pilot Study of Cognitive Intervention. J HIV AIDS Soc Serv 2004; 31: 79-97.

[32]  Mahendra N, Hopper T. Dementia and related cognitive disorders. In: Papathanasiou I, Coppens P, Potagas C, Eds. Aphasia and related neurogenic disorders. Burlington, MA: Jones & Barlett Learning 2013.

[33]  Bourgeois M. Effects of memory aids on the dyadic conversations of individuals with dementia. J Appl Behav Anal 1993; 261: 77-87.

[34]  Orsulic-Jeras S, Judge K, Camp C. Montessori- based activities for long-term are residents with advanced dementia: Effects on engagement and affect. Gerontologist 2000; 401: 107-11.

[35]  Mahendra N. Direct interventions for improving the performance of individuals with Alzheimer's disease. Semin Speech Lang 2001; 221: 291-304.

[36]  Hatakeyama R, Fukushima K, Fukuoka Y, *et al.* Personal home made digital video disk for patients with behavioral psychological symptoms of dementia. Geriatr Gerontol Int 2010; 103: 272-4.

[37]  Yasuda K, Kuwabara K, Kuwahara N, Abe S, Tetsutani N. Effectiveness of personalized reminiscence photo videos for individuals with dementia. Neuropsychol Rehabil 2009; 194: 603-19.

[38]  Groher ME. Dysphagia: Diagnosis and management. 3rd ed., Boston: Butterworth-Heinemann 1997.

[39]  Logemann JA. Evaluation and treatment of swallowing disorders. 2nd ed., Austin, TX: PRO-ED 1998.

[40]  Noll S, Bender C, Marge C. Rehabilitation of patients with swallowing disorders. In: Braddom RL, Ed. Physical Medicine and Rehabilitation. Philadelphia, Pa: WB Saunders 1996.

[41]  Paik NJ, Han TR. Critical review on the management for adult oropharyngeal dysphagia. Crit Rev Phys Rehabil Med 2002; 14: 247-72.

[42]  Drake W, O'Donoghue S, Batram C, Linday J, Greenwood R. Eating in side-lying facilitates rehabilitation in neurogenic dysphagia. Brain Inj 1997; 11: 137-42.

[43]  Welch MV, Logemann JA, Radmaker AW, Kahrilas PJ. Changes in pharyngeal dimension effected by chin tuck. Arch Phys Med Rehabil 1993; 74: 178-81.

[44]  Logemann JA, Kahrilas PJ, Kobara M, Vakil N. The benefits of head rotation on pharyngoesophageal dysphagia. Arch Phys Med Rehabil 1989; 70: 767-71.

[45]  McCulloch TM, Perlman AL, Palmer PM, Van Dale DJ. Laryngeal activity during swallow, phonation, and the Valsalva maneuver: An electromygraphic analysis. Laryngoscope 1996; 106: 1351-8.

[46]  Logemann J, Pauloski BR, Colangelo L, Lazarus C, Fujiu M, Kahrilas P. Effects of a sour bolus on oropharyngeal swallowing measures in patients with neurogenic dysphagia. J Speech Hear Res 1995; 383: 556-63.

[47]  Ylvisaker M, Logemann JA. Therapy for feeding and swallowing head injury. In: Ylvisaker M, Ed. Traumatic brain injury rehabilitation: Children and adolescents. 2nd ed. Boston, MA: Butterworth-Heinemann 1998; pp. 85-99.

[48]  Lazzara G, Lazarus C, Logemann JA. Impact on thermal stimulation on the triggering of the swallow reflex. Dysphagia 1986; 1: 73-7.

[49]  Logemann JA. Manual for the videofluroscpoic study of swallowing. 2nd ed., Austin, TX: PRO-ED 1993.

[50]  Leiter AE, Windsor J. Compliance of geriatric patients with safe-swallowing instructions. J Med Speech-Lang Pathol 1996; 8: 109-17.

[51]  Low J, Wyles C, Wilkinson T, Sainsbury R. The effect of compliance on clinical outcomes for patients with dysphagia on videofluoroscopy. Dysphagia 2001; 162: 123-7.

[52]  Crary MA, Groher ME. Introduction to adult swallowing disorders. Philadelphia, PA: Butterworth Heinemann 2003.

[53]  Macqueen E, Taubert S, Cotter D, Stevens S, Frost GS. Which commercial thickening agent do patients prefer? Dysphagia 2003; 18: 46-52.

[54]   Balasubramaniam MK, Chidambaranathan AS, Shanmugam G, Tah R. Rehabilitation of glossectomy cases with tongue prosthesis: A Literature Review. J Clin Diagn Res 2016; 102: ZE01-4.

[55]   Davis JW, Lazarus C, Logemann J, Hurst PS. Effect of a maxillary glossectomy prosthesis on articulation and swallowing. Journal of Prosthetic Density 1987; 576: 715-9.

[56]   Logemann JA, Pauloski BR, Rademaker AW, Colangeo L. Speech and swallowing rehabilitation in headand neck cancer patients. Oncology 1997; 115: 651-9.

[57]   Jordan K. Rehabilitation of the patient with dysphagia. Ear Nose Throat J 1979; 58: 86-7.

[58]   Martin BJ, Logemann JA, Shaker R, Dodds WJ. Normal laryngeal valving patterns during three breath-hold maneuvers: A pilot investigation. Dysphagia 1993; 8: 11-20.

[59]   Pouderiux P, Kahrilas PJ. Deglutitive tongue force modulation by volition, volume, and viscosity in humans. Gastroenterology 1995; 108: 1418-26.

[60]   Neumann S. Swallowing therapy with neurologic patients: Results of direct and indirect therapy methods in 66 patients suffering from neurological disorders. Dysphagia 1993; 8: 150-3.

[61]   Fujiu M, Logemann JA. Effect of a tongue-holding maneuver on posterior pharyngeal wall movement during deglutition. Am J Speech Lang Pathol 1996; 5: 25-30.

*Recent Advances in Geriatric Medicine*, 2017, Vol. 2, 123-145　　　　

## CHAPTER 9

# End of Life Care in Older Adults

Susan E. Lowey[*]

*State University of New York College at Brockport, 350 New Campus Dr, Brockport, NY 14420, USA*

**Abstract:** Older adulthood is considered to be the last phase of life in the human lifespan. According to the Centers for Disease Control and Prevention [1], the average age of death in the United States is 78 years. It is a well-known part of the human experience that death most commonly occurs during older adulthood and is more widely accepted by society than when death occurs in a child or young adult. Old age is characterized by the developmental stage of life known as integrity *versus* despair [2]. In this last developmental stage of life, an individual is left challenged to accept and find meaning in the life that he/she has lived.

**Keywords:** Death, Death and society, Dying, End of life, Family issues, Grieving, Hospice, Palliative care, Stages of development.

## INTRODUCTION

Older adults might often think more about death due to the nature of their advancing age and medical afflictions, some of which may lead to or cause death. Nonetheless, society has perceived death as a negative event and something to be feared. Discussions related to death and dying are considered taboo and avoided. Although older adults are in their last phase of life, death is still something that is often feared, not discussed and continues to be the "elephant in the room" no matter the age.

Older adults who are dying are considered to be nearing or at the end of life. The time period from the time a person is known to be dying until they die is known as *the end of life*. There is no real consensus on when the period of time known as the end of life really begins. Although it is known that the end of the end of life period commences with the death of a person, it is less clear when it really begins and how that should ideally be determined. The lack of truly being able to define

---

[*] **Corresponding author Susan E. Lowey:** State University of New York College at Brockport, 350 New Campus Dr, Brockport, NY 14420, USA; Tel: 585-395-5323; E-mail: slowey@brockport.edu

**Jeremy W. Grabbe (Ed.)**

when the end of life begins is one of the main barriers associated with providing quality end of life care. Some older adults are afflicted with illnesses in which the exact end of life period is not as clear as with other medical conditions. End of life care has been included alongside other terminology such as terminal, hospice and palliative care, and has been defined as specialized medical care that is given to a patient who is dying [3].

The length of the end of life period will vary among individuals. For some older adults, the end of life period will be shorter. Patients who suffer some type of acute trauma, such as a fall or automobile accident, or acute illness event, such as a myocardial infarction, may only have an end of life period lasting a few minutes, hours or days. For others, such as older adults who are diagnosed with heart failure or Alzheimer's disease, the end of life period can be much longer and can last several months or even years. Regardless of the length, the end of life is a time in which specialized medical care is needed in order to ease suffering and improve quality of life. The medical care that older adults receive during this time should focus on comfort rather than with the goal of curing the underlying illness. Usually by the time an older adult is considered to be at the end of life, death is anticipated and highly likely in the near future and most often the goals of medical care will ideally shift to a more comfort oriented model.

## HISTORICAL PERSPECTIVES

Historically, death usually occurred suddenly, often only days from the onset of illness. Infectious and communicable diseases such as smallpox, diphtheria and cholera were the predominant causes of death back in previous centuries [4]. The average life expectancy was much younger than in the present day, around 50 years of age [5]. The majority of deaths occurred in the home rather than the hospital with care that was provided from family members rather than health care workers. The period of time known as the end of life, was often quick with death occurring in a familiar home environment. Medical science was just beginning to develop which subsequently provided few or no options available to "save" or prolong a person's life. When someone became afflicted with an illness or infectious disease, they would die. Family members were always present witnessing much of the dying process and death of their loved one, which greatly differs from the present day. In the late 1800's and early 1900's, there was a rapid growth in the development of medicine and in the way the sick were cared for. Hospitals were being built all over the country and were now the new place where the dying went for care and died [6].

## Death in Contemporary Society

At the turn of the 20th century, significant advancements in medicine, education, and technology helped to switch the focus of care solely from providing comfort to the dying to being able to offer a partial or complete cure for many illnesses. The development of antibiotics and immunizations enabled people to become cured from many diseases that once caused certain death. The lifespan started to increase and infant mortality began to decrease, both of which are fairly good indicators about the health of a nation [5]. Chronic illnesses, such as heart disease and stroke, replaced communicable diseases as the main causes of death. In the United States today, heart disease, cancer, respiratory diseases and strokes are the top four causes of death [1]. People are often able to live many years with a chronic disease; however, it can significantly impact the overall quality of the remaining lifespan of an older adult.

Although older adults are living longer due to advances in medical science, there is also a downside. Due to the various options available to manage most illnesses, there is now difficulty in knowing when it is no longer appropriate to continue aiming for a cure. Even with the best treatment options, the natural course of disease will progress and eventually cause death. As witnessed through the news media, medical treatments are often continued beyond the point of providing benefit to the patients' life quality and instead can contribute to an increased burden and prolonged suffering.

## Illness Trajectories in End of Life Care

Although individuals each have their own unique illness experience, there are some commonalities associated with the course of various types of illnesses. Since trajectory is defined as "a course", illness trajectory can be defined as "a course of illness" and is the usual pattern or progression of an illness or disease. It is important for the health care professional who works with older adults to understand illness trajectories for several reasons. By understanding which type of illness trajectory a patient has, it will help the health care professional be able to provide answers for two important and common questions many patients have including, "how long have I got?" and "what will happen?" [7]. Older adults, and patients of any age in general, want to know what will happen to them when they are diagnosed with an illness. This is especially true if the illness is something that is not curable and the patient will have to live with that chronic illness for the rest of his/her life. The other reason that illness trajectory is an important concept health care professionals should understand is because type of trajectory can provide information as to when the patient may be nearing or at the end of life.

Each illness trajectory has its own usual course of progression and understanding that can be helpful to prepare the patient and family for what to expect and subsequently, the end of life period.

## Types of Illness Trajectories

Glaser and Strauss [8] were the first researchers who examined the various illness trajectories that people who are dying often go through. These three trajectories were referred to as: surprise deaths, expected deaths, and entry-reentry deaths. Surprise deaths are usually unexpected and occur without any prior warning, such as a motor vehicle accident. Expected deaths occur in people who are already diagnosed with some type of terminal illness and death is expected to be the outcome with disease progression. Lastly, Glaser & Strauss referred to entry-reentry deaths to describe people who have a slower illness trajectory which causes intermittent acute episodes that require hospitalization.

Since this initial classification of illness trajectories by Glaser & Strauss [8], there has been much work on this topic to further classify the most common patterns of illness progression preceding death. June Lunney and colleagues identified a four illness trajectory model found from the analysis of Medicare records of older adults who had died [9]. These trajectories include: sudden death, terminal illness, organ failure, and frailty.

Time and functional status are shown in relation to the type of illness trajectory. Sudden death is characterized by a level of high functioning with a sharp vertical decline preceding death. In this trajectory, there is no prior warning or knowledge that death will occur. The terminal illness trajectory is most common among people living with an illness that is classified as leading to terminal (*e.g.*, cancer). The person's functioning remains high throughout the illness with a rapid decline weeks or sometimes even days before death. The organ failure trajectory is quite common among many older adults living with a chronic illness that may eventually cause death. Heart failure and chronic respiratory diseases are the most common illnesses following this type of exacerbating-remitting illness progression. Although patients can bounce back from these exacerbations, there is a steady gradual decline in overall functioning over time. Lastly, the frailty trajectory depicts a long period of steady decline with very low levels of function throughout the time period. Persons with this illness trajectory often live with profound levels of disability that require maximum assistance and care for a long period of time before death. Although older adults with Alzheimer's disease can be independent in the initial part of their illness often before they are even diagnosed, this type of trajectory is what normally occurs once the patient's cognitive status declines to the point that they require assistance or dependence for all activities of daily living.

## Conversations about Goals of Care

As mentioned previously, illness trajectories can be useful in helping to assist the patient with what they might expect with illness progression. Health care professionals should initiate conversations with older adults to elicit their goals of care. Goals of care are the goals or outcomes that patients have for their individual care. They are based on patients' values and beliefs and can change over time, so it is essential that patients are asked about their goals of care periodically throughout their illness trajectory [10]. It is important to get an understanding about what the patient hopes for in terms of their illness if there is no chance for a cure. This can include whether the patient would rather focus on maintaining their quality of life even if than means a reduction in the quantity of life or time they have left. It is important to understand whether the patient would want to continue to use all medical treatments necessary to increase their lifespan even if it would make them sick. The health care professional should pose these kinds of questions to older adults so that they can begin to formulate and clarify their goals of care as they near the end of life. Older adults who may have been recently diagnosed with their illness may not have had the time or energy to think about their goals of care. In addition to the older adult, the family members may also be involved in these conversations and their own goals for the patient may differ from what the patient wants. This can be a challenge for the health care professional and team, and several family meetings may need to be held before there is resolution in a clear plan of care.

## Organized Models of End of Life Care

Many of the terms used to describe end of life care are used interchangeably and often incorrectly. Although not as widely used as in previous decades, terminal care was used to describe care given to mainly patients who were dying from an illness considered to be terminal, which was most often an end-stage cancer [3]. Comfort care is another term that is still widely used today that is defined as care used to help or soothe a person who is dying [11]. Its overall goal is to minimize suffering while maintaining the patient's wishes for the end of life. Palliative care and hospice are the two most widely recognized terms that are used to describe care that is given to older adults at the end of life. Both modes of care operate under the same philosophical idea, which is to provide comfort for the patient by focusing on palliating symptoms. They do, however, differ in terms of specific admission requirements and are used differently within the larger health care system. Regardless of the term, the goal of all of these types of care given at the end of life to those is to prevent and relieve suffering while trying to maintain the person's wishes and goals of care.

## Palliative Care

Palliative care is derived from the term "palliate" which is to reduce the violence of (a disease) and/or to ease (symptoms) without curing the underlying disease. Palliative care has also been further defined by the World Health Organization as an approach to care that improves the quality of life for patients with life-limiting illnesses and their families through the prevention and relief of physical, psychosocial and spiritual suffering [12]. Palliative care is not only the underlying philosophy of most organized end of life care programs, such as hospice, but also its own specialty of care. Currently in the United States, over half of all 100-plus bed hospitals have a palliative care program and in hospital palliative care programs have increased by 138% since the beginning of this century [13].

Palliative care uses a team-based approach to evaluate and manage the various effects of any illness that can cause distress. Most often comprised of physicians, mid-level providers, and nurses, in-hospital palliative care teams evaluate hospitalized patients who need better symptom management and/or have been recently diagnosed with a terminal illness and need assistance with decision making and care planning. Older adults living with a serious illness often have pain or other symptoms that decrease their overall quality of life and contribute to suffering. Palliative care clinicians also provide emotional support for patients and their families to help them during this difficult time in their lives.

Palliative care can be used with patients of any age or any stage of illness because the overarching goal is to improve quality of life [13]. Unlike hospice care, there is no pre-determined life expectancy required to be eligible or to receive palliative care. Over the past few years several sub-specialties of palliative care have been developed including geriatric and pediatric palliative care, which focuses on improving quality of life in specialized populations, such as with older adults and children. According to the End of Life Nursing Education Consortium (ELNEC), palliative care services are often paid for through fee-for-service, philanthropy, or through direct hospital support [14].

## Hospice Care

The term "hospice" was first coined during the medieval period and was considered to be a place where weary travelers could rest [15]. Hospice is one type of formal end of life care delivery system that is supported by reimbursement from Medicare and many of the major health insurance carriers. According to the National Hospice and Palliative Care Organization (NHPCO), the focus of hospice is on caring for instead of curing a patient's terminal illness. Hospice originated from the United Kingdom with the first U.S. hospice opening in 1971. Since then, hospice programs have steadily grown and by 2012, there were approximately 5,500 hospice programs in the U.S [15]. Fifty-seven percent of patients received hospice in a free-standing hospice, 20% in a hospital, 17% from a home health agency, and 5% from a nursing home according to NHPCO.

Hospice care was originally developed for patients with a terminal diagnosis of cancer, so many of its rules and regulations fit the care needs of the oncology population well. Over the past decade, the rate of hospice use among non-cancer diagnoses has significantly increased. Patients with cancer diagnoses accounted for only 36.9% of all hospice admissions, whereas the remaining 63.1% of admissions were patients with non-cancer illnesses [15]. Heart disease, dementia and debility were found to be the most common non-cancer illnesses of patients admitted to hospice care [15]. In order to quality for hospice care, patient's need to have an estimated life expectancy of 6 months or less as certified by a physician.

Similar to palliative care, hospice also uses a team approach that consists of a physician, nurse and social worker, in the least. Patients admitted to hospice elect one primary physician to oversee their medical care. Reimbursement for hospice can include the following services: (a) Physician services, (b) Nursing care, (c) Medical equipment & supplies related to terminal illness, (d) Medications for management of pain and other symptoms related to terminal illness, (e) Hospice care aide services, (f) Physical and occupational therapy, (g) Social work services (h) Dietary counseling, (i) Spiritual counseling and (j) Bereavement care [16].

Since the focus of hospice care is pursuing comfort rather than cure, part of the hospice requirements is that patients forgo any curative life-sustaining medical treatments and instead only receive care that is aimed at improving quality of life. This can be initially difficult for patients and families to understand but often fall in line with the patient's overall goals of care. The following are some of the services that hospice reimbursement does not cover: (a) Inpatient hospitalizations for life-sustaining treatments (b) Diagnostic interventions such as x-rays or lab work, (c) Emergency room care, (d) Care from a specialist aimed at curative measures, (e) Some types of outpatient services and (f) Ambulance services (Centers for Medicare & Medicaid Services, 2013). Many older adults often do not want to go back to the hospital for treatments and would rather stay at home to receive care.

### Similarities and Differences between Hospice and Palliative Care

Hospice and palliative care are the two most widely used formal end of life care programs in the United States. Both modes of care provide special care and support for individuals living with serious illnesses through an interdisciplinary team approach. They both focus on improving quality of life through interventions that provide comfort and reduce the negative effects caused by the terminal illness. Lastly, both programs support both the patient who is living with the terminal illness and their family who is caring for them.

One of the main differences between hospice and palliative care is the timing of when care can be initiated. Palliative care can be given at any age and any stage of a person's illness trajectory and should ideally be instituted alongside curative care when a person is first diagnosed with a serious illness. This differs from hospice care, which is only initiated for individuals who have a life expectancy of less than 6 months as certified by their physician and for whom curative medical treatments are no longer an option or are desired by the patient (NHPCO, 2013). The other main difference between hospice and palliative care are the rules governing the use of curative *versus* comfort care. Hospice requires that patients forgo all medical treatments that are life-sustaining or curative in nature and elect to receive care that only focused on providing comfort. This differs from palliative care in which patients are able to receive life-sustaining or curative treatments right alongside palliative care.

For many older adults who are afflicted with chronic advanced illnesses such as heart failure or chronic obstructive pulmonary disease, the various rules governing what hospice care does or does not allow, may not be consistent with the goals of care for these patients. For example, patients with heart failure have exacerbations of their illness that often require hospitalization and administration of medications that are considered as being curative. These patients would have to forgo these interventions if electing to make the switch to hospice care. Although hospice is a widely used and well received care program for patients at the end of life, it may not provide the care desired by patients with certain diagnoses, such as heart failure, whose measures used for symptom management are considered curative and would not be reimbursable through the hospice benefit.

## Management of Pain & Symptoms at the End of Life

As older adults are nearing the end of life, they often have some distressing symptoms related to their advancing illness that can greatly impact their quality of life. As mentioned at the beginning of this chapter, older adults who are diagnosed with an illness often have many questions and concerns not only about their prognosis but also about what their illness will bring as it becomes more advanced or end stage [17]. As illnesses progress to a terminal state, there can be one or more physical manifestations of discomfort. The dying process can affect the physiological, psychological or emotional and spiritual health of older adults. It is important for health care professionals to evaluate their patients for the presence of symptoms or concerns related to each of these facets of health so that early and rapid management can be implemented. It is especially important to note that the focus of end of life care is as much on non-physiological concerns as is physical pain and symptoms, as to those affected; the dying process is much more than just the cessation of body processes.

### Physiological Health

Patients that are dying experience a wide range of symptoms, with pain as one of the most prevalent, particularly with older adults who have cancer [18]. Shortness of breath or breathlessness is another common and distressing symptom that occurs at the end of life in patients who have heart failure or chronic pulmonary disease. Additionally, older adults nearing the end of life can also experience symptoms such as: cough, nausea and vomiting, constipation, diarrhea, anorexia and cachexia, dysphagia, fatigue, seizures, lymphedema, depression, anxiety and terminal delirium. We will now discuss several of the most common symptoms that occur in older adults at the end of life.

### *Pain*

Older adults can experience and express their physical pain very differently [18]. Pain perceptions can vary according medical diagnosis, cognitive functioning, cultural background and other factors. Individuals will report pain differently and health professionals should evaluate other expressions of discomfort as possible indicators for pain, such as reductions in activity level or appetite, new or worsening depression, withdrawal from social situations, and problems with sleep.

Pain is classified by its physiological origin (somatic, visceral, or neuropathic) and also by its pattern of presentation (acute or chronic) [19]. The first step in pain assessment is to understand what type of pain the patient is presenting with in order to be able to utilize the best intervention to treat it. Nociceptive pain, which is also known as somatic, is pain that is well localized to one area of the body. An example of this is bone pain. Visceral pain is another type of pain that is described as a deep squeezing or pressure that is not as well localized to one area of the body. This type of pain often results from some type of compression or stretching of thoracic or abdominal viscera. An example of this would be pain that accompanies pancreatic or liver cancer [19]. Neuropathic pain is associated with an illness or injury to the peripheral or central nervous system and is described as is described as a sharp, shooting, or burning pain. Patient's that have a tumor pressing on a specific nerve or an illness that affects the nerves experience this type of pain [19].

Older adults should be asked about their current location of pain, its intensity, quality, aggravating factors, alleviating factors, duration, and current pain management regimen [14]. Once the specific type and origin of pain is determined, the health care provider will be able to tailor the pain management plan to meet the needs of the patient. Pain management can include both pharmacological and non-pharmacological measures. Short lived acute pain is often managed by use of a short-acting analgesic whereas chronic pain management often includes the use of both a long-acting and short-acting analgesic medications [14]. Due to the various aging related changes in older adults, pain medications should be used according to the World Health Organization (WHO) three-step ladder for pain in adults [20]. Pain should always be treated with the lowest type of analgesia that will reduce the pain and limit unwanted side effects. This is especially important with older adults due to the unique pharmacokinetics in this population. The risk of side effects is greater in older adults however, adequate pain assessment and management should be used and pain treated appropriately Narcotic analgesic medications may contribute to falls, delirium, urinary retention and other effects and should be used alongside non-narcotic medications, which may help reduce the dosage of the narcotic medication [21].

### Shortness of Breath

Shortness of breath or breathlessness is a common physiological process associated with the dying process. It has been described by patients as feeling as if they were struggling to breathe and not able to get enough air. It is a frightening experience and can contribute to increased levels of anxiety [14]. When some illnesses become end-stage, dyspnea or shortness of breath, becomes refractory.

This means that the underlying cause cannot be reversed and the focus of care must shift to interventions aimed at palliation [22]. Since the causes of shortness of breath can be multidimensional, effective management of this symptom can be challenging. Currently the gold standard management for refractory dyspnea in end of life care is the use of an opioid medication [23]. Again, in older adults, use of narcotics should be closely monitored however in older adults who are actively dying; the benefits of the treatment may outweigh the burden since the focus is on improving their quality of life.

## *Anorexia & Cachexia*

Anorexia and cachexia are two common issues that arise in older adults at the end of life. Depending on the type of illness an older adult is diagnosed with, anorexia may be a symptom that he/she has dealt with throughout the course of illness. Anorexia is defined as a loss of appetite and/or lack of desire to eat which causes reduced caloric intake [14]. The lack of adequate nutrition can lead to a syndrome known as cachexia which is defined as wasting away from lack of adequate nutrition [14]. Weight loss is the presenting feature in both anorexia and cachexia and is often difficult to treat in patients nearing the end of life.

Discussions related to the use of artificial nutrition and hydration are often a result from the presence of anorexia and cachexia. This is one of the most distressing issues that family members of older adults at the end of life go through. Although it is difficult to witness your loved one wasting away, health care professionals should educate patients and families on the dying process and the benefits and burdens associated with artificial hydration and nutrition. The evidence has shown that most often artificial nutrition and hydration is contraindicated in patients at the end of life. This is because it has been found to be more of a burden than benefit and can lead to the development or worsening of nausea and vomiting, edema or shortness of breath [14]. Appetite stimulants, such as Megestrol, may also be used to help boost appetite but each individual patient must be evaluated to see if this would be an appropriate measure to use [21].

## *Terminal Delirium*

Delirium is a common occurrence at the end of life that is frequently under-diagnosed and poorly managed [24]. The presentation of terminal delirium is not that different from regular delirium in patients, however terminal delirium or restlessness only occurs in patients who are dying and at the end of life [14]. As with older adults in general, delirium is commonly mistaken for dementia and is a probable reason for why it is under-diagnosed [21]. The key sign is that delirium has an abrupt onset with changes in consciousness and cognition which may fluctuate throughout the day [24]. Terminal delirium occurs in nearly 90% of patients who are nearing death [14].

Older adults nearing the end of life often have metabolic or endocrine disturbances that are irreversible and therefore interventions should be aimed at supporting the patient and family and providing pharmacological treatment to decrease symptoms. The presence of spiritual distress can also contribute to terminal restlessness or delirium in some patients with unresolved issues [14]. It is important to provide a quiet and peaceful environment for the patient which can help ease symptoms. Aromatherapy has been shown to provide a calming effect in some patients [24]. Pharmacological management includes the use of haloperidol as the primary medication used to treat terminal restlessness/delirium. Benzodiazepines may also be used but may precipitate a worsening effect, particularly in elderly patients [14].

**Psychological Health**

There is a large focus in end of life care on the management of physiological pain and symptoms. While this is important, older adults who are dying also experience psychological and emotional distress that is often less frequently discussed or evaluated. Patients who are at the end of life feel loss and grief about their impending death and often go through a progression of stages throughout this process. Dr. Elisabeth Kuebler Ross classified how individuals who are dying cope [25]. The five stages that were identified include: denial, anger, bargaining, depression, and acceptance. Not all older adults who are dying will go through each of these stages in this order or may not reach all of these stages at all.

*Denial*

This is the first stage because this is how older adults will initially react to being told that they have a poor prognosis and limited time. Patients are often in disbelief and may not believe what they have been told by their physician. Some patients may get a second opinion from another physician during this stage. Denial can be beneficial for the patient initially as it acts as a shock absorber which can enable them to internalize and begin to process that information.

*Anger*

In the second stage, older adults have processed that their impending death is true and they are angry about it. Patients in this stage are making the realization that their time is not limited and they may not be able to accomplish some of the things they wanted to. They may be angry at their physician or other care providers and their family. It is important for health professionals to support the family during this stage and to tell them that their loved one is experiencing normal feelings and that their anger is at their illness situation and not the family.

## Bargaining

Bargaining is the third stage is called and it happens internally with the person who is dying. Patients at this stage may bargain with a higher power to change their outcome and give them more time. Some patients may try to bargain with their physician for other options that could prolong their death.

## Depression

Feelings of depression can be a normal reaction for patients who are dying. They are upset because they may have had things they wanted to accomplish and that are now being cut short. At this time, patients may be physically declining in health, losing some functioning, and experiencing increased symptoms.

## Acceptance

The last stage is acceptance. During this stage, patients have come to terms with their impending death and have found a sense of internal peace. The preceding stages have led to negative emotions and now that some time has progressed, patients can begin to move past the shock and anger about their situation and focus on the time they have left. During this stage, their hope for a cure is often replaced by a hope that their end of life will be as peaceful and pain free as possible.

## Spiritual Health

Patients who are dying often think about their own spirituality. The end of life is a time when some people become more in touch with their own spirituality. The knowledge of impending death can make people embrace, strengthen and re-ignite their spiritual health. For others, they may not want to discuss their spirituality and may feel anger at their situation and angry at higher powers they feel are responsible for their impending death. Unresolved or distressing spiritual issues at the end of life can be just as important for patients as unmanaged pain and should be considered to be a priority by healthcare professionals. The role of healthcare professionals and spiritual care has been found to go beyond the realm of a specific or prescribed "role" and instead is a highly interpersonal process that is embedded in the context of the human experience [26]. Being present and really opening one's eyes to the patient's individual situation were identified in this study as important facilitators of spiritual care. Health care professionals can provide spiritual support and if comfortable, even pray with their patient. Lack of time in the health care setting or encounter was identified as a barrier to providing good spiritual care. Identification of whether a patient wants to speak to a Chaplain or member of the clergy is important to evaluate in older adults at the end of life, particularly if the healthcare clinician perceives time to be a barrier in their individual care setting.

## Ethical Challenges at the End of Life

Ethical issues and challenges can arise when patients and families engage in medical decision making related to the care they want or do not want as they near the end of life. Many of these decisions are difficult and contribute to distress and feelings of guilt among family members who are often left to make these choices on behalf of the patient. These decisions can be related to the types of medical treatments that they do or do not wish to have, the timing about when to stop receiving certain medical interventions, whether certain life sustaining measures are desired and who should be elected to speak on behalf of the patient when he/she is no longer able. It is not uncommon for conflicts to arise between the various participants who are involved in these decisions, including the patient, their family, the provider, and the health care system.

### *Resuscitation and Advance Directives*

According to the Patients' Rights Council [27], an advance directive is a document that states the medical care a patient wants in the event that they can no longer make their own decisions. A living will and a durable power of attorney for health care are two types of advance directives that an older adult can execute in the event they are not able to engage in their medical decisions.

### *Do Not Resuscitate (DNR)*

In the past decade, the American Heart Association has added a different terminology used to describe a patient's resuscitation status. Previously, the acronym (DNR) was used for do-not-resuscitate, which meant that a patient did not want any medical intervention if they went into cardiopulmonary arrest. Another acronym (DNAR), do-not-attempt resuscitation, has recently been added. This acronym is being used in some medical facilities as a less harsh term to denote the decision for not medically intervening when a patient goes into cardiac arrest. If a patient has an order for a DNR or DNAR, it means that the patient has elected for cardiopulmonary resuscitation (CPR) to not be initiated or administered in the event of a cardiac arrest. CPR could include the use of chest compressions, cardiac drugs and the placement of a breathing tube.

Older adults with serious illnesses often have poor outcomes when CPR is used. Berry & Griffie [28] found that CPR was successful for only about 18% of hospitalized patients who have arrested over the past 50 years. The success rate percentage has found to be even lower among patients with advanced terminal illnesses, such as cancer or end stage heart failure. Older adults commonly have one or more co-morbidities that contribute to the low success rate of CPR. A do-not-intubate (DNI) order, often accompanies a DNR/DNAR order. A DNI order states that the patient does not wish to be intubated with a breathing tube if they go into cardiac arrest. Other resuscitation interventions, such as chest compressions and the use of cardiac medications could still be used, depending on the patient's advance directive.

### *Allow Natural Death (AND)*

Allow natural death is another term being used by some health care institutions in place of the traditional DNR/DNAR. An AND order states that only comfort measures should be taken to manage any symptoms in a patient who is expected to die [14]. The goal of an AND order is to enable the patient to remain comfortable while not interfering with the natural process of dying that he/she is going through.

### *Medical Order for Life Sustaining Treatment (MOLST)*

Sometimes also referred to as physician order to life-sustaining treatment (POLST), these newer forms of advance directives, were developed to improve the communication between healthcare providers and settings regarding a patient's wishes about life sustaining interventions. The MOLST/POLST is currently being used in 26 states across the United States (POLST Organization, 2014).

### *Withholding and Withdrawing Care*

Medical interventions used at the end of life can range from minor, such as the use of a non-life sustaining medication, to complex, such as mechanical ventilation. One of the all too common dilemmas that occur in patients at the end of life relates to stopping certain medical interventions in patients. The medical interventions that are stopped, or in some cases, never initiated, are interventions aimed at curative medical care. Interventions for comfort and palliative care continue to be provided. The rationale behind the cessation of these curative interventions is often based on evaluating the burdens against any benefits from these treatments. Some types of life-sustaining therapies can prolong suffering and decrease the patient's quality of life. Patients and their family often decide to stop medical interventions based on their goals of care.

One of the most difficult decisions that family members have to make pertains to withdrawing life sustaining care or life support, from their loved ones. This is why having medical wishes known in advance is so important. As mentioned previously, advance directives are documents that enable patients to make their decisions about medical care known to their family and health care providers, in the event that they are unable to make those decisions themselves [29]. Knowing a patient's wishes and carrying out those wishes can help to alleviate some of the burden family members may feel about making these decisions. By knowing what a patient wants ahead of time, it can help prevent the initiation of select life sustaining treatments beforehand. It is often easier to not initiate life sustaining treatments initially rather than making the decision to withdraw that intervention at some later date. Advance directives can help to decreased futile medical care [30].

### Artificial Nutrition and Hydration

A common concern at the end of life is about the use of artificial nutrition or hydration (ANH). ANH is defined as an intervention that delivers nutrition and/or hydration through artificial means. It usually involves administering food or fluids through non oral means, through subcutaneous or intravenous means [31]. According to the American Hospice Foundation, the use of ANH should be considered no more than basic care rather than a medical treatment [31]. Although this is not the case as its use, or lack thereof, poses ethical concern at the end of life. Previous research has determined that food and mealtime is symbolic and the act of not being able to provide food or fluids to our loved ones is distressing [32]. However, the research has suggested that patients who are dying actually derive some benefit from not eating or drinking such as decreased nausea, shortness of breath and edema [32]. This research has found that many physicians view ANH as "standard care" that is lacking any empirical support. Most families do not want to have their loves one "starve to death", however, have difficulty withholding ANH if it is offered as an option by providers. This is one of those issues that impede the natural course of disease through intervening by artificial means. More research is needed in this very challenging emotion driven issue in end of life care.

## Grief and Bereavement

Grief and bereavement are universal experiences that people go through when they are dealing with a loss in their lives. We often equate loss in terms of a human being, such as a family member or friend. However, loss can include the loss of independence, functional ability and cognitive status as faced by thousands of older adults each day. Those non-human losses can also precipitate feelings of grief. Grief and bereavement are important concepts for the health care professional to understand in the context of end of life care because they can have negative effects that should be evaluated in patients and families who are facing the end of life.

### What is Grief?

Grief is an emotional response to a loss and is often a process that occurs before the death of a loved one who is facing the end of life [14]. Older adults who know they have a life limiting condition can grieve as they anticipate the future to come. They often go through a process, similar to the states of dying, that can help them progress to coping with their impending death. This process has been referred to as "grief work" and as with the stages of dying, people can progress through these stages differently. Family members also go through these stages as they learn to cope with the eventual loss of their loved one [14].

Corless [33] developed a three-stage grief framework that includes these three components: (a) notification and shock, (b) experience the loss, and (c) reintegration. The initial stage is when the individual first learns about the loss. Feelings of shock may ensue and they often isolate themselves from others during this first stage. The second stage is characterized by fully experiencing the loss on an emotional and cognitive level. Feelings of anger, emptiness, and sadness can occur. Individuals will also sometimes have physical manifestations of the loss, such as insomnia, loss of appetite or headaches. The last stage is characterized by a re-organization and re-integration of a new life without their loved one who has died. Ideally, healing should be the end result to occur by this final third stage in this model. Certainly, not everyone will follow this framework but it characterizes the main components of how many individuals deal with loss. Health care professionals should understand that individuals will experience loss in unique ways; however, manifestations of grief can proceed to abnormal behaviors and feelings that could impede the healing process. This is when interventions should be offered for the bereaved.

## *Types of Grief*

Individuals can express a variety of grief reactions towards a loss. There can be a range of reactions that fluctuate by varying degrees between normal and abnormal and that can occur both before and after a loss.

### *Normal or Uncomplicated Grief*

Normal or uncomplicated grief symbolizes the most desirable and universal reaction that can be expected following a loss [33]. A normal reaction to the loss can include physical, emotional, cognitive, and behavioral reactions immediately following the loss that will eventually progress to adjustment. The time that an individual will progress to adjusting or coping with the loss varies from person to person and is dependent on the type of relationship and type of loss that occurred.

### *Anticipatory Grief*

Grief that occurs before the loss of a loved one is common among patients and their family members who are facing the end of life. Anticipatory grief can begin at the time of a terminal diagnosis and can proceed until death occurs. Both the patient and family can go through anticipatory grief. Patients often anticipate their loss of independence, physical or cognitive functioning and comfort. This can be very distressing for the patient who is experiencing it. Family members who have a loved one who is expected to die often start the grieving process early when they initially learn that their loved one will die. This type of grief has been shown to be protective and cushion an individual's bereavement reaction [33].

### *Complicated Grief*

Complicated grief is an abnormal grief reaction that may require professional assistance depending on severity [14]. Individuals who experience sudden or traumatic losses, such as those resulting from suicide/homicide, can be at risk for complicated grief reactions. Individuals who have gone through multiple losses or recent losses which have not been resolved can also be at greater risk for developing complicated grief reactions. Additionally, the lack of a support system or concurrent stressors such as health, relationship or financial issues also can contribute to this type of grief [14].

Complicated grief can be further classified into four different types which include: (a) chronic grief, (b) delayed grief, (c) exaggerated grief, and (d) masked grief. Chronic grief is characterized by normal grief reactions that continue for longer extended periods of time. Delayed grief reactions are normal grief reactions that are suppressed due to a conscious or unconscious avoidance of feelings of loss. Exaggerated grief is marked by an intense reaction to the loss that can be accompanies by nightmares, the development or worsening of phobias, and also can include suicidal thoughts. Lastly, masked grief reactions are characterized by behaviors that the individual does not attribute to their recent loss [14].

## *Disenfranchised Grief*

Grief that has not been validated or recognized is called disenfranchised grief [14]. Individuals who have lost loved ones to stigmatized illnesses, such as AIDS or through socially unacceptable ways, such as abortion, are at risk for experiencing this type of grief reaction. The loss of a previously severed relationship, such as what often takes place with divorce, can also put individuals at greater risk. This is because the individual often has to mourn privately due to the circumstances surrounding the severed relationship.

## *Unresolved Grief*

In unresolved grief, the individual has failed to move through the stages of grief and accomplish the work needed to come to terms with the loss, therefore the grief is said to be unresolved [33]. The lack of formal closure, multiple or concurrent losses, or social isolation are risk factors that can precipitate this grief reaction.

## ***Manifestations of Grief***

Grief can be expressed in terms of physical, emotional, cognitive, and behavioral reactions to the loss. The bereaved individual can feel pain from their loss in any or all of these ways. Common physical manifestations of grief include: general ill feeling, headaches, heaviness or pressure in the chest or stomach, tremors, muscle aches, exhaustion and insomnia. Cognitive manifestations may include: inability to concentrate, feelings of confusion or disbelief, pre-occupation with the deceased and hallucinatory experiences. Emotional manifestations can include: anxiety, guilt, anger, sadness, feelings of helplessness, and relief. Common behavioral manifestations include: withdrawal, impaired performance at work or school, avoidance behaviors and/or possessing constant reminders of the deceased [14].

## ***Bereavement***

Bereavement is defined as the "time period in which the survivor adjusts to their life without their loved one" [14]. This period can include both grief and mourning and is characterized by the time following the loss or death, the funeral, and during the grieving process that follows. Factors such as age, physical and emotional health, culture, and previous experience with loss/death can all affect the way a person adjusts during this period of time. Bereavement differs from grief in that it includes the period of time from the beginning of the loss until acceptance has been reached. Mourning also occurs during this time period and can differ based on personal and cultural factors.

## Letting Go

Letting go, has been a concept that has been explored in the context of death and dying [17, 34]. Family members caring for a loved one during the dying process often experience this phenomenon of letting go. Letting go has been described as a process in which the end result is recognition and acceptance of the impending death. The acceptance has been said to be a freedom from the immense emotional experiences that were experienced prior to letting go. This can occur both before the death and after and can be part of the grief and bereavement process. Lowey [17] conducted a concept analysis of 'letting go' and found four distinct attributes that compose the concept. These include: (1) a shift in thinking, or a crucial turning point, (2) recognition that despite efforts to save their loved one, they are dying or have died and all hope for recovery or prolonged life is exhausted, (3) acknowledgment of the impending physical and emotional loss that will occur with the death and (4) allowing the progression to inevitable death to occur by choosing not to prolong or impede its natural progression. Some of these attributes are similar to anticipatory grief, anticipatory mourning and death awareness.

## **Support during Bereavement**

Bereaved individuals can use both informal and formal supports to help them deal with the loss of their loved one. The kind of support an individual will need differs and part of end of life care can include a formal grief assessment. ELNEC [14] recommends that assessment of grief occur at regular intervals throughout the course of illness and should initially occur at diagnosis. Grief should be assessed frequently during the bereavement period so that an effective plan can be developed for the bereaved in coping with their loss. Most hospice programs offer formal bereavement services and events to promote closure and acceptance. An example of this is the implementation of memorial services to honor recent patients who have died. Both family members and staff alike are invited to participate in the memorial services which can be effective at helping both parties find closure. Many communities and/or health care systems offer various support groups for individuals, some of which are specific to a particular type of illness (*i.e.* cancer). Individual or group counseling are other methods that can assist the bereaved in coping with their loss.

## CONCLUSION

End of life issues contain a myriad of factors. These factors can range from the patient's needs and desires to comfort and support for loved ones. Assessment at the end of life can be confounded by medical and psychological influences on the patient's well-being. The modern approach is to understand the steps/stages associated with end of life and provide specific support.

## CONFLICT OF INTEREST

The author confirms that author has no conflict of interest to declare for this publication.

## ACKNOWLEDGEMENTS

Declared none.

## REFERENCES

[1]     Centers for Disease Control and Prevention. Leading causes of death 2015. Available from: http://www.cdc.gov/nchs/fastats/leading-causes-of-death.htm.

[2]     Erikson E. Childhood and society. 2nd ed., New York, N.Y.: Norton 1963.

[3]     Izumi S, Nagae H, Sakurai C, Imamura E. Defining end-of-life care from perspectives of nursing ethics. Nurs Ethics 2012; 19(5): 608-18.
        [http://dx.doi.org/10.1177/0969733011436205] [PMID: 22990423]

[4]     Judd D, Sitzman K, Davis GM. A history of American nursing: Trends and eras. Sudbury, MA: Jones & Bartlett 2010.

[5]     Stanhope M, Lancaster J. Foundations of nursing in the community: Community oriented practice. 4th ed., St. Louis, MO: Mosby Elsevier 2014.

[6]     Reverby SM. Ordered to care: The dilemma of American nursing, 1850-1945. Cambridge, UK: Cambridge University Press 1987.

[7]     Murray SA, Kendall M, Boyd K, Sheikh A. Illness trajectories and palliative care. BMJ 2005; 330(7498): 1007-11.
        [http://dx.doi.org/10.1136/bmj.330.7498.1007] [PMID: 15860828]

[8]     Glaser BG, Strauss AL. Awareness of dying. New Brunswick: AldineTransaction 1965.

[9]     Lunney JR, Lynn J, Hogan C. Profiles of older medicare decedents. J Am Geriatr Soc 2002; 50(6): 1108-12.
        [http://dx.doi.org/10.1046/j.1532-5415.2002.50268.x] [PMID: 12110073]

[10]    Vermont Ethics Network. Palliative care and pain management: Importance of goals for care 2011. Available from: http://www.vtethicsnetwork.org/importance_of_goals.html.

[11]   U.S. Department of Health and Human Services, National Institute on Aging. End of life: Helping with comfort and care (NIH Publication No 08-6036) 2012. Available from: https://www.nia.nih.gov/health/publication/end-life-helping-comfort-and-care/introduction.

[12]   World Health Organization. WHO definition of palliative care 2014. Available from: http://www.who.int/cancer/palliative/definition/en/.

[13]   Center to Advance Palliative Care. Building a palliative care program 2011. Available from: http://www.capc.org/building-a-hospital-based-palliative-care-program/.

[14]   End of Life Nursing Education Consortium ELNEC - core curriculum training program. City of Hope and American Association of Colleges of Nursing 2010. Available from: http://www.aacn.nche.edu/ELNEC.

[15]   National Hospice and Palliative Care Organization. Hospice and palliative care 2014. Available from: http://www.nhpco.org/about/hospice-care.

[16]   Centers for Medicare & Medicaid Services. Medicare hospice benefits 2013. Available from: http://www.medicare.gov/pubs/pdf/02154.pdf.

[17]   Lowey SE. Letting go before a death: a concept analysis. J Adv Nurs 2008; 63(2): 208-15.
[http://dx.doi.org/10.1111/j.1365-2648.2008.04696.x] [PMID: 18544043]

[18]   McPherson CJ, Hadjistavropoulos T, Lobchuk MM, Kilgour KN. Cancer-related pain in older adults receiving palliative care: patient and family caregiver perspectives on the experience of pain. Pain Res Manag 2013; 18(6): 293-300.
[http://dx.doi.org/10.1155/2013/439594] [PMID: 23957019]

[19]   Coyle N, Layman-Goldstein M. Pain assessment and management in palliative care. In: LaPorte-Matzo M, Witt-Sherman D, Eds. Palliative Care Nursing: Quality Care to the End of Life. New York: Springer 2001; pp. 362-486.

[20]   World Health Organization. WHO's cancer pain ladder for adults 1990. Available from: http://www.who.int/cancer/palliative/painladder/en/.

[21]   Eliopoulos C. Gerontological nursing. 8th ed., Philadelphia, PA: Wolter Kluwer Health 2014.

[22]   Abernethy AP, Currow DC, Frith P, Fazekas BS, McHugh A, Bui C. Randomised, double blind, placebo controlled crossover trial of sustained release morphine for the management of refractory dyspnoea. BMJ 2003; 327(7414): 523-8.
[http://dx.doi.org/10.1136/bmj.327.7414.523] [PMID: 12958109]

[23]   Lanken PN, Terry PB, Delisser HM, *et al*. An official American Thoracic Society clinical policy statement: palliative care for patients with respiratory diseases and critical illnesses. Am J Respir Crit Care Med 2008; 177(8): 912-27.
[http://dx.doi.org/10.1164/rccm.200605-587ST] [PMID: 18390964]

[24]   Heidrich DE, English N. Delirium, confusion, agitation, and restlessness. In: Ferrell BR, Coyle N, Eds. Oxford textbook of palliative nursing. New York: Oxford University Press 2010; pp. 449-68.
[http://dx.doi.org/10.1093/med/9780195391343.003.0022]

[25]   Kuebler-Ross E. On Death and Dying. New York: Scriber Publishing Group 1997.

[26]   Daaleman TP, Usher BM, Williams SW, Rawlings J, Hanson LC. An exploratory study of spiritual care at the end of life. Ann Fam Med 2008; 6(5): 406-11.
[http://dx.doi.org/10.1370/afm.883] [PMID: 18779544]

[27]   Patients Rights Council. Advance directives: Definitions 2013. Available from: http://www.patients-rightscouncil.org/site/advance-directives-definitions/.

[28]    Berry P, Griffie J. Planning for the actual death. In: Ferrell BR, Coyle N, Eds. Oxford Textbook of Palliative Nursing. New York: Oxford University Press 2010; pp. 629-44.
[http://dx.doi.org/10.1093/med/9780195391343.003.0033]

[29]    National Cancer Institute. Facts sheets: Advance directives 2013. Available from: http://www.cancer. gov/cancertopics/factsheet/Support/advance-directives.

[30]    Coyne PJ, Smith TJ, Lyckholm LJ. Oxford textbook of palliative nursing. New York: Oxford University Press 2010; pp. 487-99.
[http://dx.doi.org/10.1093/med/9780195391343.003.0025]

[31]    Arenella C. Artificial nutrition and hydration at the end of life: Beneficial or harmful? Available from: https://americanhospice.org/caregiving/artificial-nutrition-and-hydration-at-the-end-of-life-beneficial-or-harmful/.

[32]    Brody H, Hermer LD, Scott LD, Grumbles LL, Kutac JE, McCammon SD. Artificial nutrition and hydration: the evolution of ethics, evidence, and policy. J Gen Intern Med 2011; 26(9): 1053-8.
[http://dx.doi.org/10.1007/s11606-011-1659-z] [PMID: 21380599]

[33]    Corless IB. Bereavement. In: Ferrell BR, Coyle N, Eds. Oxford textbook of palliative nursing. New York: Oxford University Press 2010; pp. 597-611.
[http://dx.doi.org/10.1093/med/9780195391343.003.0031]

[34]    Zerwekh JV. Nursing care at the end of life: Palliative care for patients and families. Philadelphia, PA: F.A. Davis Company 2006.

# SUBJECT INDEX